The Ultimate Mediterranean Diet Cookbook

Delicious Breakfast Recipes To Burn Fat And Promote Longevity

Ben Cooper

© Copyright 2020 - All rights reserved.

The content contained within this book may not be reproduced, duplicated or transmitted without direct written permission from the author or the publisher.

Under no circumstances will any blame or legal responsibility be held against the publisher, or author, for any damages, reparation, or monetary loss due to the information contained within this book. Either directly or indirectly.

Legal Notice:

This book is copyright protected. This book is only for personal use. You cannot amend, distribute, sell, use, quote or paraphrase any part, or the content within this book, without the consent of the author or publisher.

Disclaimer Notice:

Please note the information contained within this document is for educational and entertainment purposes only. All effort has been executed to present accurate, up to date, and reliable, complete information. No warranties of any kind are declared or implied. Readers acknowledge that the author is not engaging in the rendering of legal, financial, medical or professional advice. The content within this book has been derived from various sources. Please consult a licensed professional before attempting any techniques outlined in this book. By reading this document, the reader agrees that under no circumstances is the author responsible for any losses, direct or indirect, which are incurred as a result of the use of information contained within this document, including, but not limited to, — errors, omissions, or inaccuracies.

Table of contents

Bacon and Brussels Sprout Breakfast 7

Mushroom & Spinach Omelet 9

Cheesy Yogurt 13

Artichokes and Cheese Omelet 15

Walnut Poached Eggs 17

Almond Cream Cheese Bake 19

Chili Egg Cups 21

Dill Eggs Mix 23

Hummus and Tomato Sandwich 25

Buttery Pancakes 27

Cream Olive Muffins 29

Herbed Fried Eggs 31

Chili Scramble 33

Couscous and Chickpeas Bowls 35

Anti-inflammatory blueberry smoothie 37

Cherry - Pomegranate Smoothie Bow - Gluten-Free & Vegetarian 39

Breakfast Banana Green Smoothie 41

Strawberry Oatmeal Breakfast Smoothie 43

Kale and Banana Smoothie 45

Pumpkin pie fall smoothie 47

Green Tart Smoothie 49

Gluten-free pancakes 51

Crunchy quinoa meal 53

Coconut pancakes 55

Quinoa porridge	57
Banana Barley Porridge	61
Zucchini Muffins	63
Millet Porridge	65
Jackfruit Vegetable Fry	67
Zucchini Pancakes	69
Squash Hash	71
Pumpkin Spice Quinoa	73
Sweet Cashew Cheese Spread	75
Mini Zucchini Bites	77
Beef with broccoli on cauliflower rice	79
Asparagus & crabmeat frittata	82
Bacon cheeseburger	85
Cheeseburger Pie	88
Ancho tilapia on cauliflower rice	79
Multigrain blueberry yogurt pancakes	90
Mediterranean Frittata	92
Banana Blueberry Muffins	94
Spiced chickpeas bowls	97
Avocado Spread	99
Baked omelet mix	101
Veggie Bowls	103
Mediterranean egg cup	105
Avocado and Apple Smoothie	107

Bacon and Brussels Sprout Breakfast

Preparation Time: 10 minutes
Cooking Time: 15 minutes
Servings: 3

Ingredients:

Apple cider vinegar, 1½ tbsps.
Salt
Minced shallots
2 Minced garlic cloves
2 Medium eggs
3 Sliced Brussels sprouts
12 oz. Black pepper
Chopped bacon, 2 oz
Melted butter, 1 tbsp

Directions:

1. Over medium heat, quick fry the bacon until crispy then reserve on a plate

2. Set the pan on fire again to fry garlic and shallots for 30 seconds
Stir in apple cider vinegar, Brussels sprouts, and seasoning to cook for five minutes

3. Add the bacon to cook for five minutes then stir in the butter and set a hole at the center

4. Crash the eggs to the pan and let cook fully
Enjoy

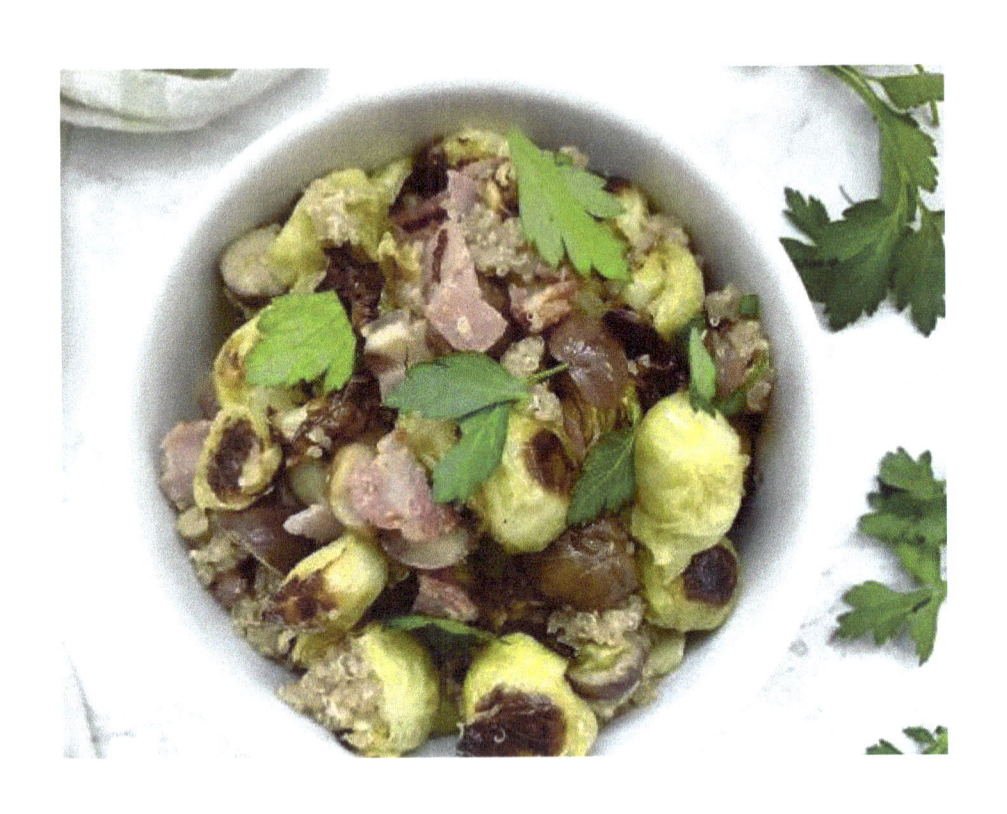

Mushroom & Spinach Omelet

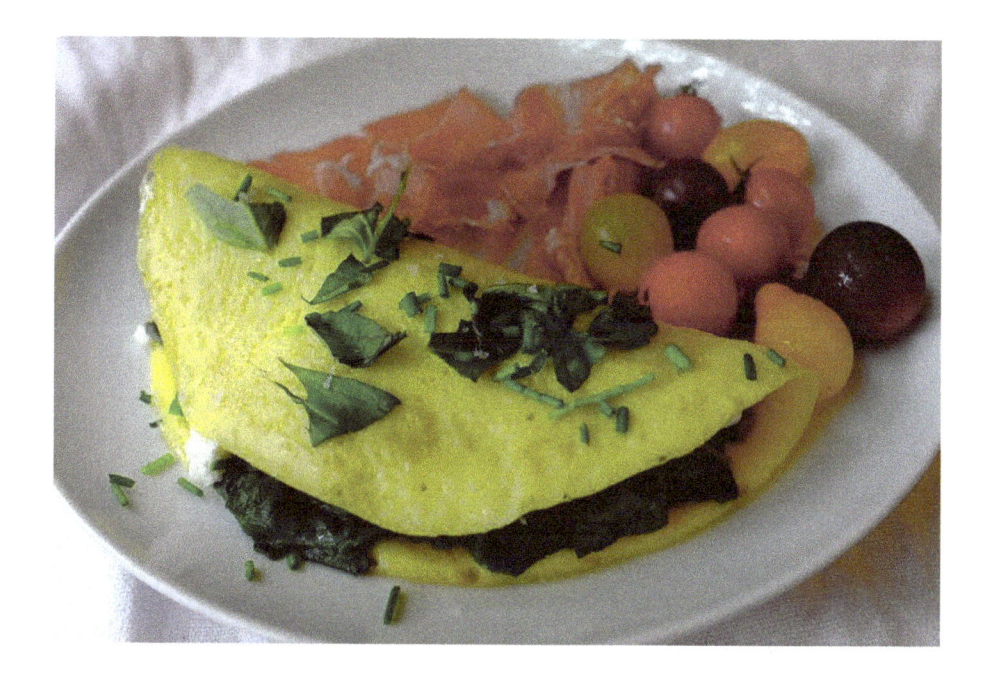

Preparation Time: 20 minutes

Cooking Time: 20 minutes

Servings: 3

Ingredients:

2 tablespoons butter divided

6-8 fresh mushrooms, sliced

5 ounces Chives, chopped, optional
Salt and pepper, to taste

1 handful baby spinach

About 1/2 ounce Pinch garlic powder

4 eggs, beaten

1-ounce shredded Swiss cheese

Directions:

1.In a very large saucepan, sauté the mushrooms in one tablespoon of butter until soft. Season with salt, pepper, and garlic.

2.Remove the mushrooms from the pan and keep warm. Heat the remaining tablespoon of butter in the same skillet over medium heat.

3.Beat the eggs with a little salt and pepper and add to the hot butter.

4Turn the pan over to coat the entire bottom of the pan with egg. Once the egg is almost out, place the cheese over the middle of the tortilla.

5.Fill the cheese with spinach leaves and hot mushrooms. Let cook for about a minute for the spinach to start to wilt. Fold the tortilla's empty side carefully over the filling and slide it onto a plate and sprinkle with chives, if desired.

6.Alternatively, you can make two tortillas using half the mushroom, spinach, and cheese filling in each.

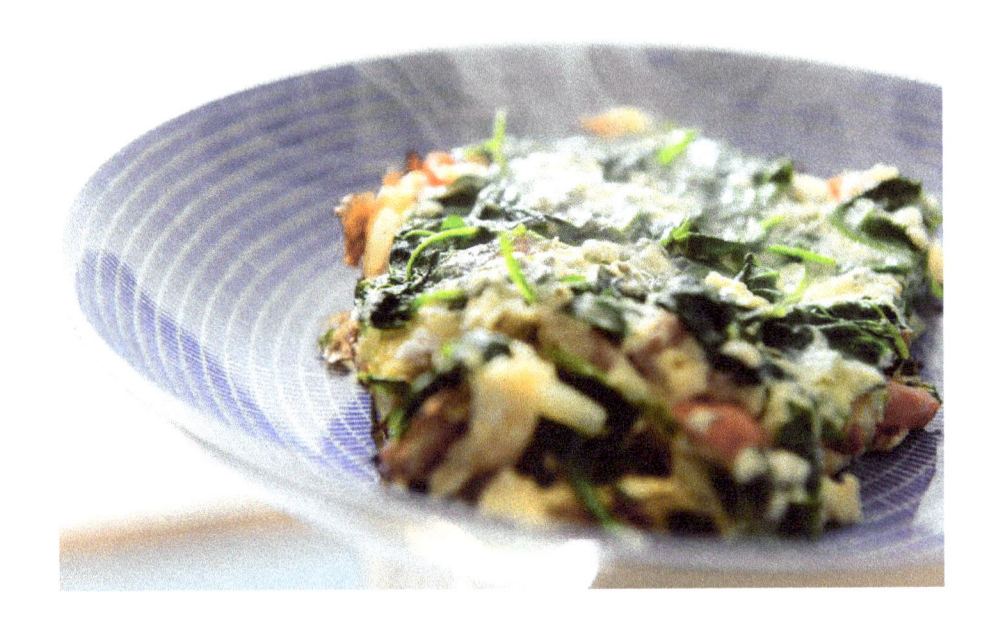

Cheesy Yogurt

Preparation Time: 4 hours and 5 minutes
Cooking Time: 0 minutes
Servings: 4

Ingredients:
1 cup Greek yogurt 1 tbsp. honey
½ cup feta cheese, crumbled

Directions:

1.In a blender, combine the yogurt with the honey and the cheese and pulse well.

2. Divide into bowls and freeze for 4 hours before serving for breakfast.

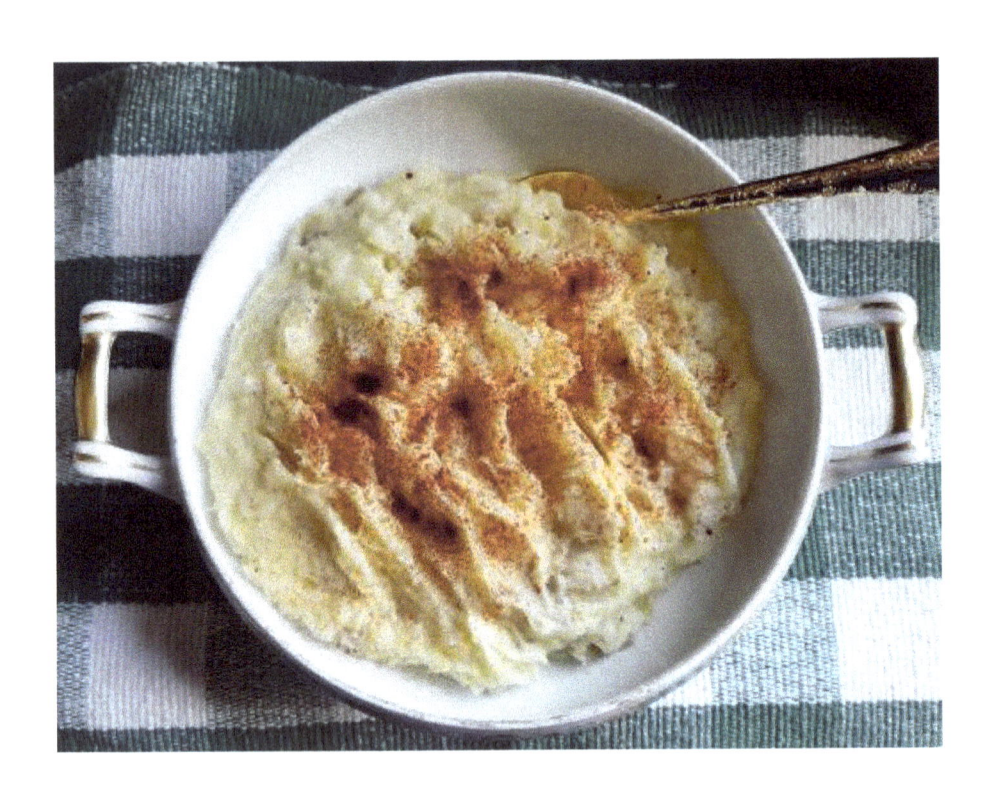

Artichokes and Cheese Omelet

Preparation Time: 10 minutes Cooking Time: 8 minutes Servings: 1
Ingredients:

1 tsp. avocado oil
1 tbsp. almond milk 2 eggs, whisked
A pinch of salt and black pepper 2 tbsp. tomato, cubed
2 tbsp. kalamata olives, pitted and sliced 1 artichoke heart, chopped
1 tbsp. tomato sauce
1 tbsp. feta cheese, crumbled

Directions:

1. In a bowl, combine the eggs with the milk, salt, pepper and the rest of the ingredients except the avocado oil and whisk well.

2. Heat a pan with the avocado oil over medium-high heat, add the omelet mix, spread into the pan, cook for 4 minutes, flip, cook for 4 minutes more, transfer to a plate and serve.

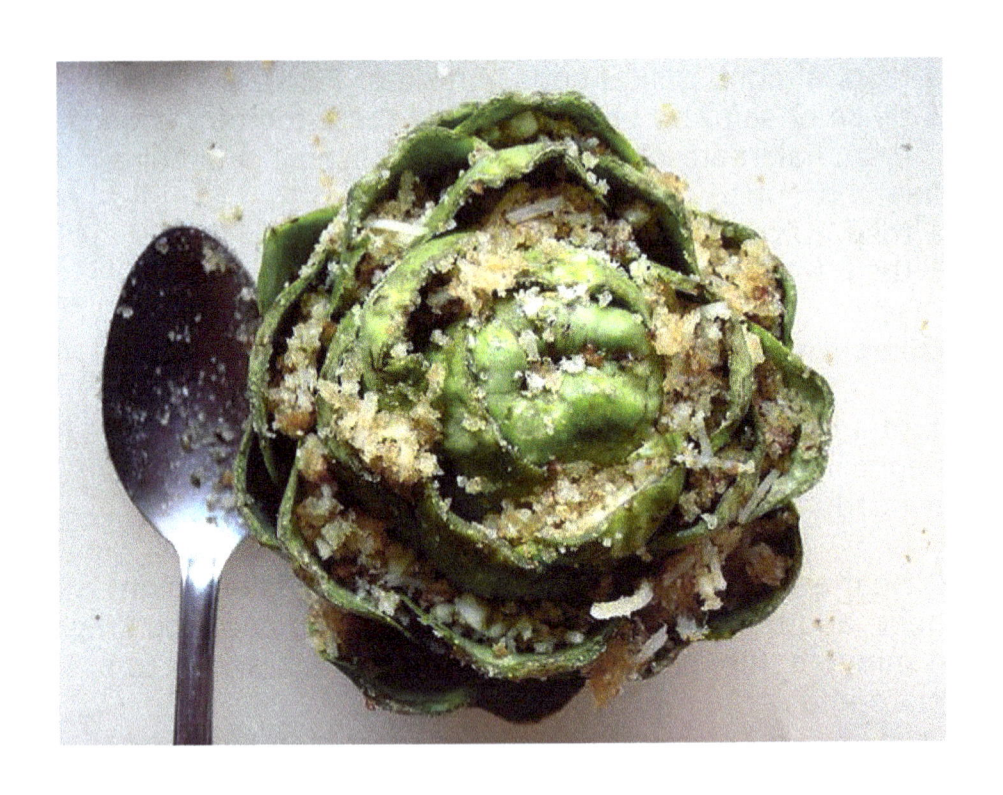

Walnut Poached Eggs

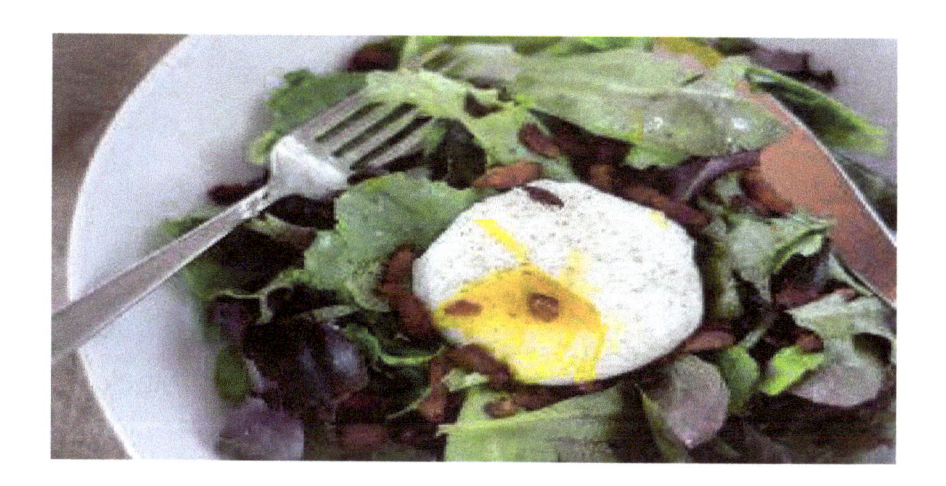

Preparation Time: 10 minutes
Cooking Time: 10 minutes
Servings: 2

Ingredients:

2 slices whole grain bread toasted 1 oz sun-dried tomato, sliced
1 tbsp. cream cheese 1/3 tsp. minced garlic 2 slices prosciutto
2 eggs 1 tbsp. walnuts
½ cup fresh basil
1 oz Parmesan, grated 3 tbsp. olive oil
¼ tsp. ground black pepper 1 cup water, for cooking

Directions:

1. Pour water in the saucepan and bring it to boil.

2. Then crack eggs in the boiling water and cook them for 3-4 minutes or until the egg whites are white.

3. Meanwhile, churn together minced garlic and cream cheese.

4. Spread the bread slices with the cream cheese mixture.

5. Top them with the sun-dried tomatoes.

6. Make the pesto sauce: Blend together ground black pepper, Parmesan, olive oil, and basil. When the mixture is homogenous, pesto is cooked.

7. Carefully transfer the poached eggs over the sun-dried tomatoes and sprinkle with pesto sauce.

8. The poached eggs should be hot while serving.

Almond Cream Cheese Bake

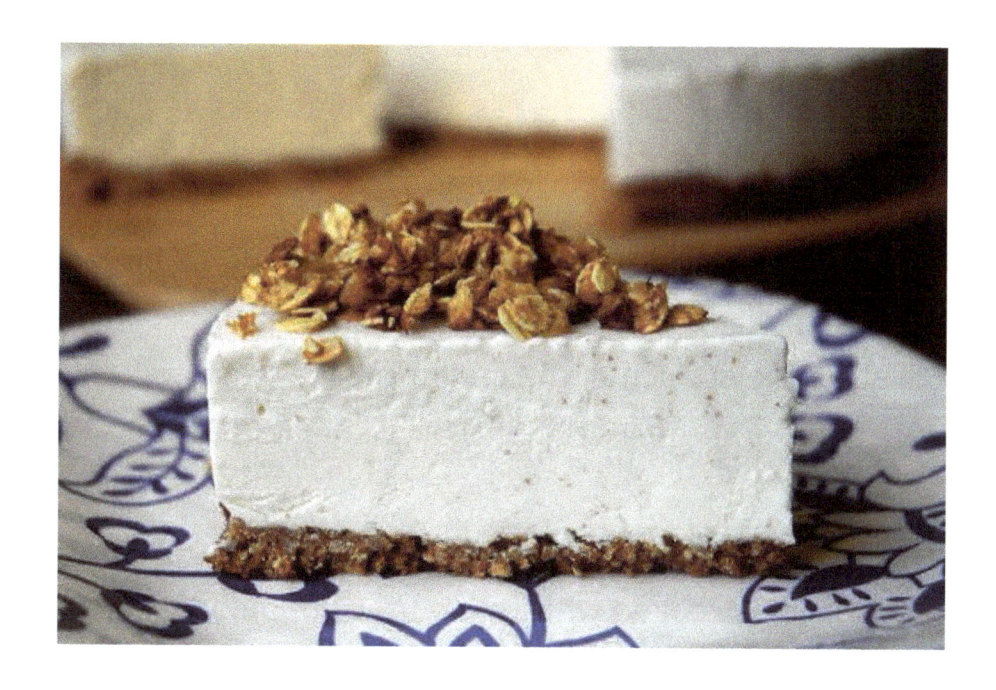

**Preparation Time: 10 minutes
Cooking Time: 2 hours
Servings: 4**

Ingredients:
1 cup cream cheese 4 tbsp
honey 1 oz almonds, chopped
½ tsp. vanilla extract
3 eggs, beaten
1 tbsp semolina

Directions:

1. Put beaten eggs in the mixing bowl.

2.Add cream cheese, semolina, and vanilla extract.

3.Blend the mixture with the help of the hand mixer until it is fluffy.

4.After this, add chopped almonds and mix up the mass well.

5.Transfer the cream cheese mash in the non-sticky baking mold.

6.Flatten the surface of the cream cheese mash well.

7.Preheat the oven to 325°F.

8.Cook the breakfast for 2 hours.

9.The meal is cooked when the surface of the mash is light brown.
10.Chill the cream cheese mash little and sprinkle with honey.

Chili Egg Cups

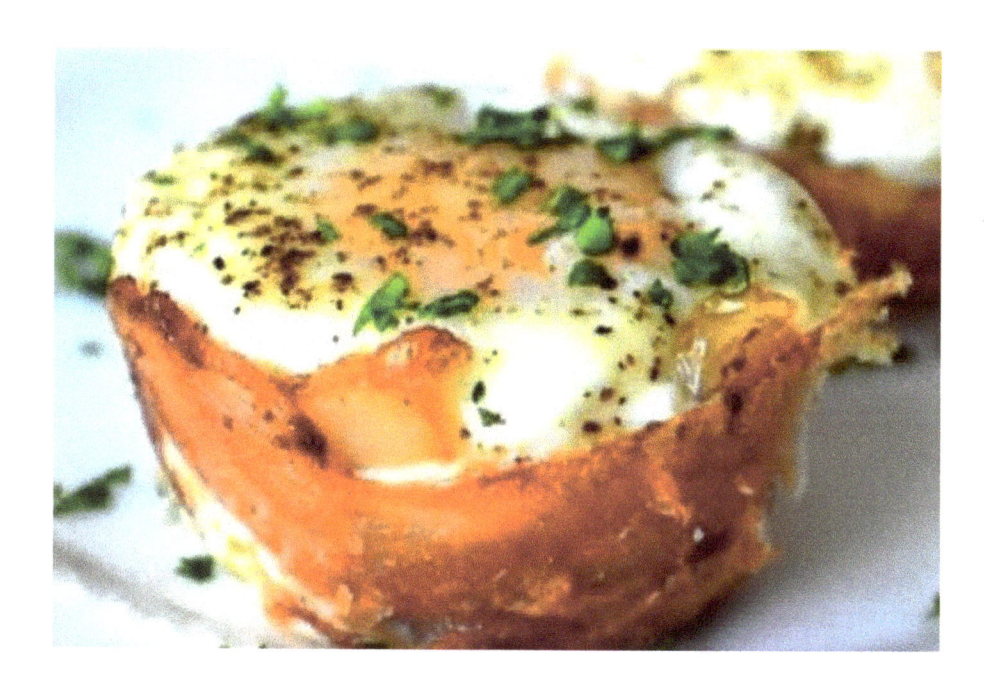

Preparation Time: 15 minutes
Cooking Time: 15 minutes
Servings: 4

Ingredients:
1 tsp. chives, chopped 4 eggs
1 tsp. tomato paste 1 tbsp. Plain yogurt
½ tsp. butter, softened
¼ tsp. chili flakes
½ oz Cheddar cheese, shredded

Directions:

1. Preheat the oven to 365°F.

2.Brush the muffin molds with the softened butter from inside.

3.Then mix up together Plain yogurt with chili flakes and tomato paste.

4.Crack the eggs in the muffin molds.

5.After this, carefully place the tomato paste mixture over the eggs and top with Cheddar cheese.

6.Sprinkle the eggs with chili flakes and place in the preheated oven.

7.Cook the egg cups for 15 minutes.

8.Then check if the eggs are solid and remove them from the oven.
10.Chill the egg cups till the room temperature and gently remove from the muffin molds.

Dill Eggs Mix

Preparation Time: 10 minutes
Cooking Time: 15 minutes
Servings: 2

Ingredients:
2 eggs
2 oz Feta cheese
1 tsp. fresh dill, chopped 1 tsp. butter
½ tsp. olive oil
¼ tsp. onion powder
¼ tsp. chili flakes

Directions:

1. Toss butter in the skillet.

2. Add olive oil and bring to boil.

3. After this, crack the eggs in the skillet.

4. Sprinkle them with chili flakes and onion powder.

5. Then preheat the oven to 360°F.

6. Transfer the skillet with eggs in the oven and cook for 10 minutes.

7. Then crumble Feta cheese and sprinkle it over the eggs.

8. Bake the eggs for 5 minutes more.

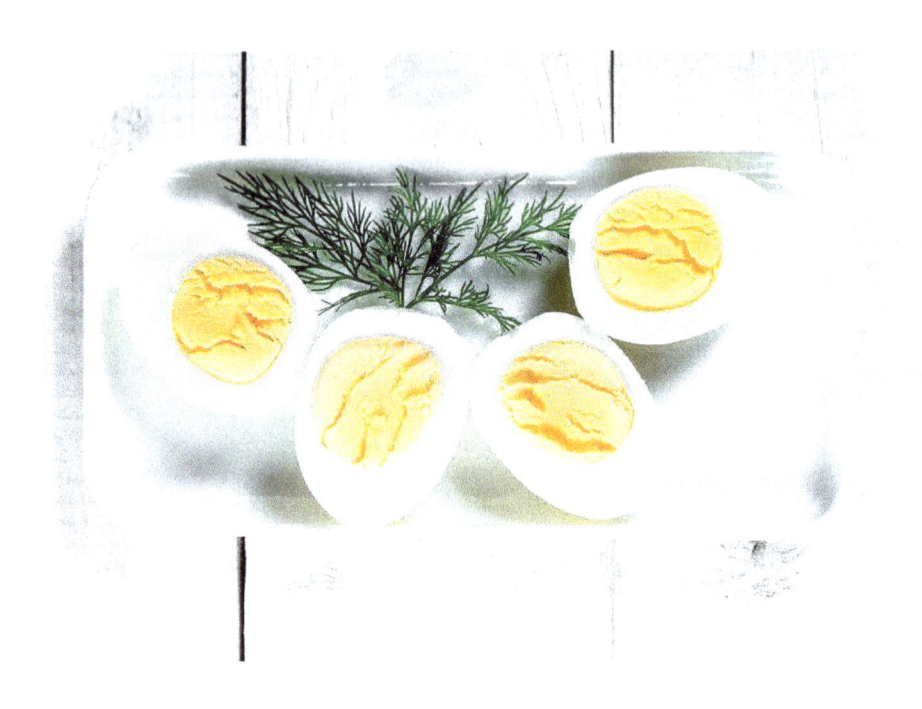

Hummus and Tomato Sandwich

Preparation Time: 10 minutes
Cooking Time: 2 minutes
Servings: 3

Ingredients:

6 whole grain bread slices 1 tomato
3 Cheddar cheese slices
½ tsp. dried oregano
1 tsp. green chili paste
½ red onion, sliced 1 tsp. lemon juice 1 tbsp. hummus
3 lettuce leaves

Directions:

1. Slice tomato into 6 slices.

2. In the shallow bowl mix up together dried oregano, green chili paste, lemon juice, and hummus.

3. Spread 3 bread slices with the chili paste mixture.

4. After this, place the sliced tomatoes on them.

5. Add sliced onion, Cheddar cheese, and lettuce leaves.

6. Cover the lettuce leaves with the remaining bread slices to get the sandwiches.

7. Preheat the grill to 365°F.

8. Grill the sandwiches for 2 minutes.

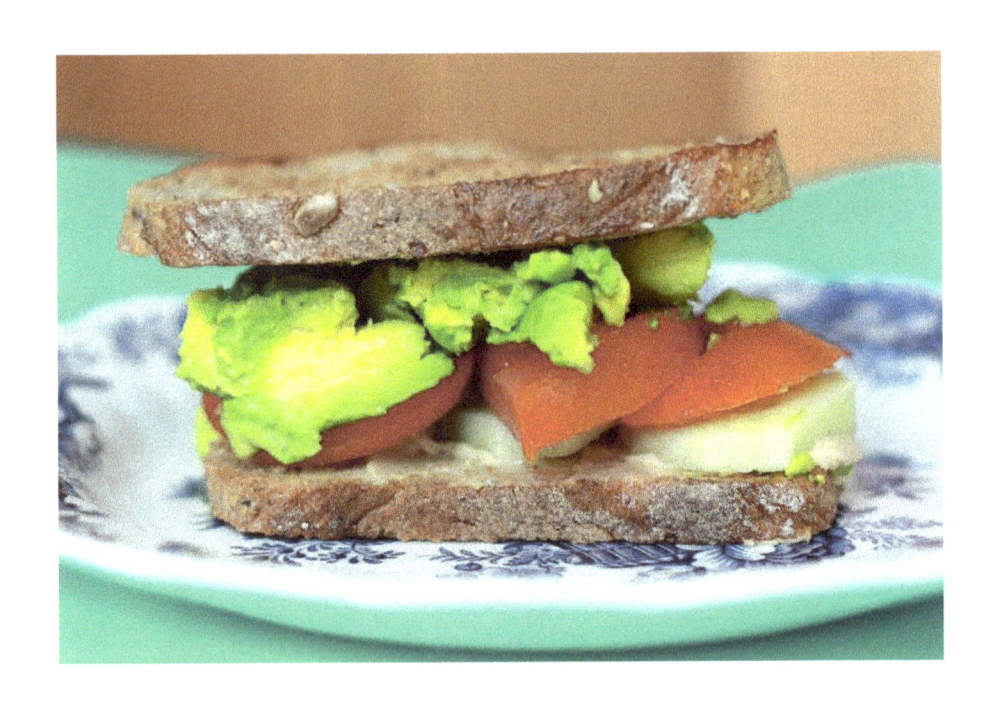

Buttery Pancakes

Preparation Time: 10 minutes
Cooking Time: 10 minutes
Servings: 5

Ingredients
1 cup wheat flour, whole-grain 1 tsp. baking powder
1 tsp. lemon juice 3 eggs, beaten
¼ cup Splenda
1 tsp. vanilla extract 1/3 cup blueberries 1 tbsp. olive oil
1 tsp. butter 1/3 cup milk

Directions:

1. In the mixer bowl, combine baking powder, wheat flour, lemon juice, eggs, Splenda, vanilla extract, milk, and olive oil.

2. Blend the liquid until it is smooth and homogenous.

3. After this, toss the butter in the skillet and melt it.

4. With the spoon's help pour the pancake batter in the hot skillet and flatten it in the shape of the pancake.

5. Sprinkle the pancake with the blueberries gently and cook for 1.5 minutes over the medium heat.

6. Then flip the pancake onto another side and cook it for 30 seconds more.

7. Repeat the same steps with all remaining batter and blueberries.

8.Transfer the cooked pancakes in the serving plate.

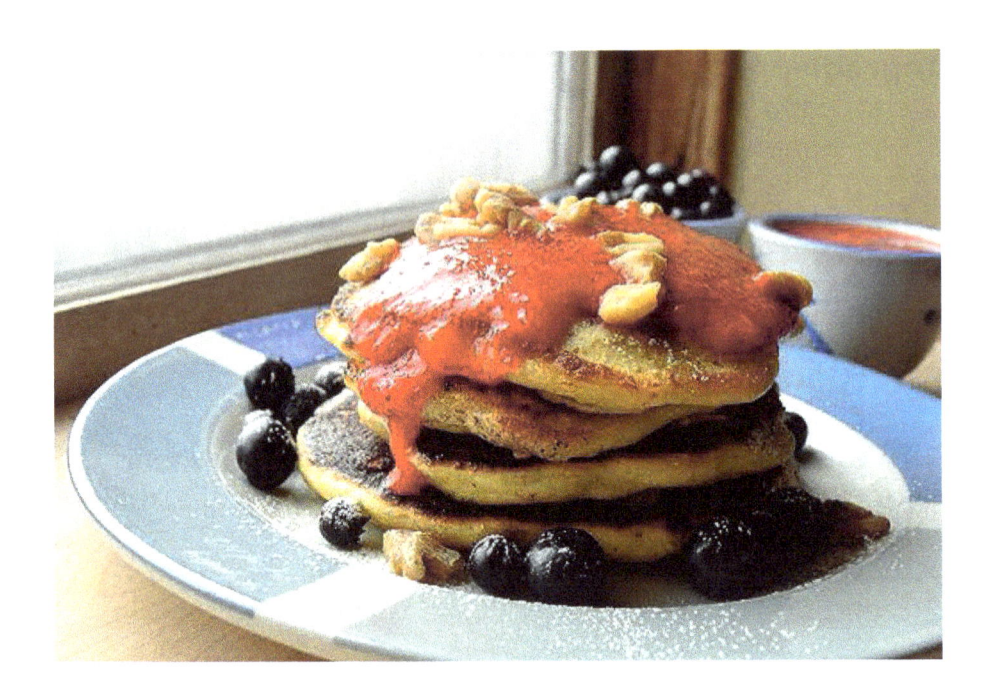

Cream Olive Muffins

Preparation Time: 15 minutes
Cooking Time: 20 minutes
Servings: 6

Ingredients:

½ cup quinoa, cooked
2 oz Feta cheese, crumbled 2 eggs, beaten
3 kalamata olives, chopped
¾ cup heavy cream 1 tomato, chopped
1 tsp. butter, softened
1 tbsp. wheat flour, whole grain
½ tsp. salt

Directions:

1. In the mixing bowl whisk eggs and add Feta cheese.

2. Then add chopped tomato and heavy cream.

3. After this, add wheat flour, salt, and quinoa.

4. Then add kalamata olives and mix up the ingredients with the help of the spoon.

5. Brush the muffin molds with the butter from inside.

6. Transfer quinoa mixture in the muffin molds and flatten it with the spatula or spoon's help if needed.

7. Cook the muffins in the preheated to 355°F oven for 20 minutes.

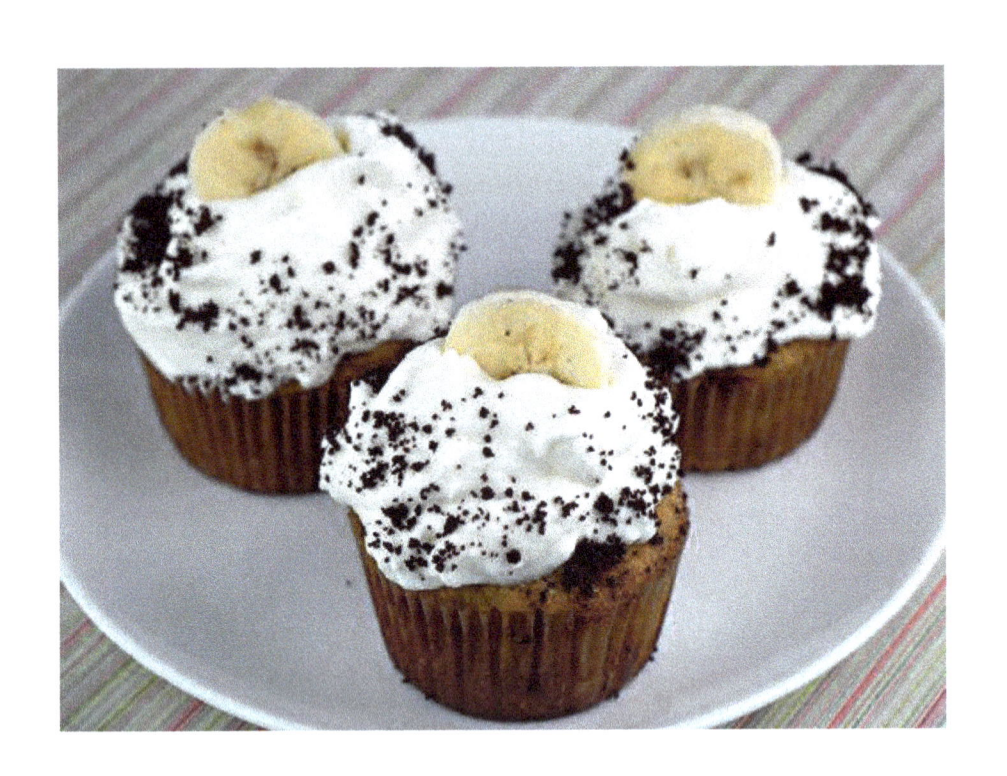

Herbed Fried Eggs

Preparation Time: 6 minutes
Cooking Time: 7 minutes
Servings: 2

Ingredients:
4 eggs
1 tbsp. butter
½ tsp. chives, chopped
½ tsp. fresh parsley, chopped 1/3 tsp. fresh dill, chopped
¾ tsp. sea salt

Directions:

1. Toss butter in the skillet and bring it to boil.

2. Then crack the eggs in the coiled butter and sprinkle with sea salt.

3. Cook the eggs with the closed lid for 2 minutes over the medium heat.

4. Then open the lid and sprinkle them with parsley, dill, and chives.

5. Cook the eggs for 3 minutes more over the medium heat.

6. Carefully transfer the cooked meal in the plate. Use the wooden spatula for this step.

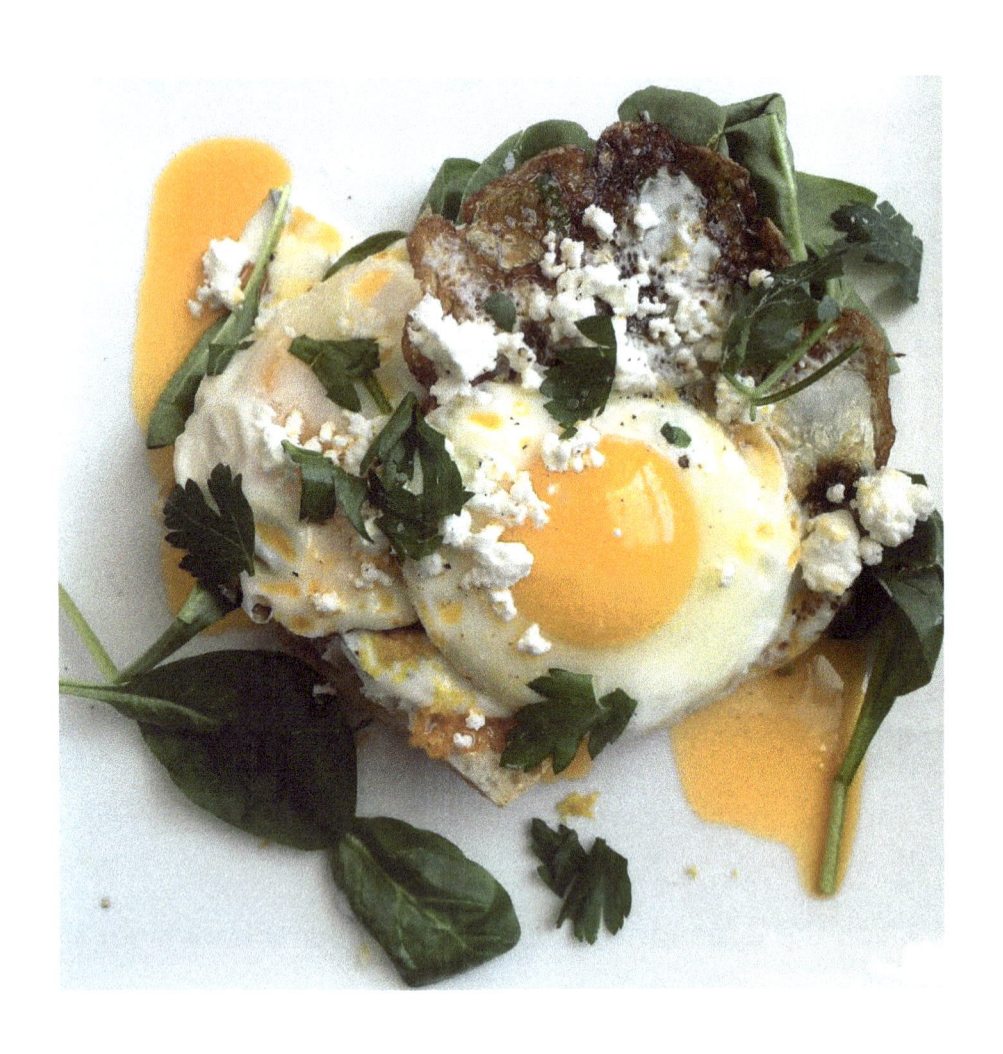

Chili Scramble

Preparation Time: 15 minutes
Cooking Time: 15 minutes
Servings: 4

Ingredients:
3 tomatoes
4 eggs
¼ tsp. of sea salt
½ chili pepper, chopped 1 tbsp. butter
1 cup water, for cooking

Directions:

1. Pour water in the saucepan and bring it to boil.

2. Then remove water from the heat and add tomatoes.

3. Let the tomatoes stay in the hot water for 2-3 minutes.

4. After this, remove the tomatoes from water and peel them.

5. Place butter in theee pan and melt it.

6. Add chopped chili pepper and fry it for 3 minutes over the medium heat.

7. Then chop the peeled tomatoes and add into the chili peppers.

8. Cook the vegetables for 5 minutes over the medium heat. Stir them from time to time.

9.After this, add sea salt and crack the eggs

10.Stir (scramble) the eggs well with the fork's help and cook them for 3 minutes over the medium heat.

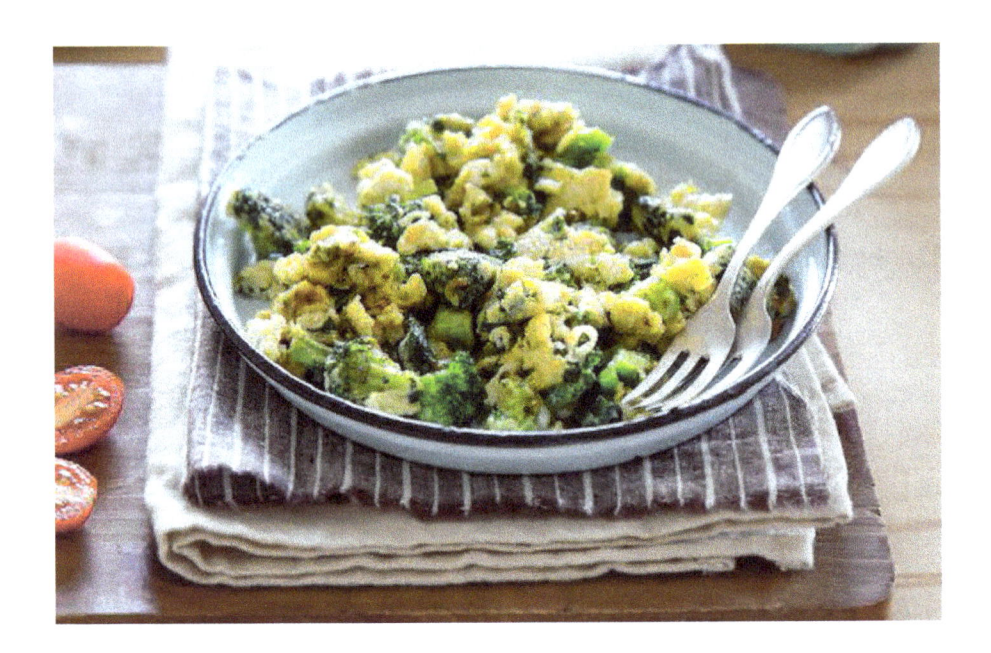

Couscous and Chickpeas Bowls

Preparation Time: 10 minutes
Cooking Time: 6 minutes
Servings: 4

Ingredients:
¾ cup whole wheat couscous 1 yellow onion, chopped
1 tbsp. olive oil 1 cup water
2 garlic cloves, minced
15 oz. canned chickpeas, drained and rinsed A pinch of salt and black pepper
15 oz. canned tomatoes, chopped
14 oz. canned artichokes, drained and chopped
½ cup Greek olives, pitted and chopped
½ tsp. oregano, dried 1 tbsp. lemon juice

Directions:

1.Put the water in a pot, bring to a boil over medium heat, add the couscous, stir, take off the heat, cover the pan, leave aside for 10 minutes and fluff with a fork.

2.Heat a pan with the oil over medium-high heat, add the onion and sauté for 2 minutes.

3.Add the rest of the ingredients, toss and cook for 4 minutes more.

4.Add the couscous, toss, divide into bowls and serve for breakfast.

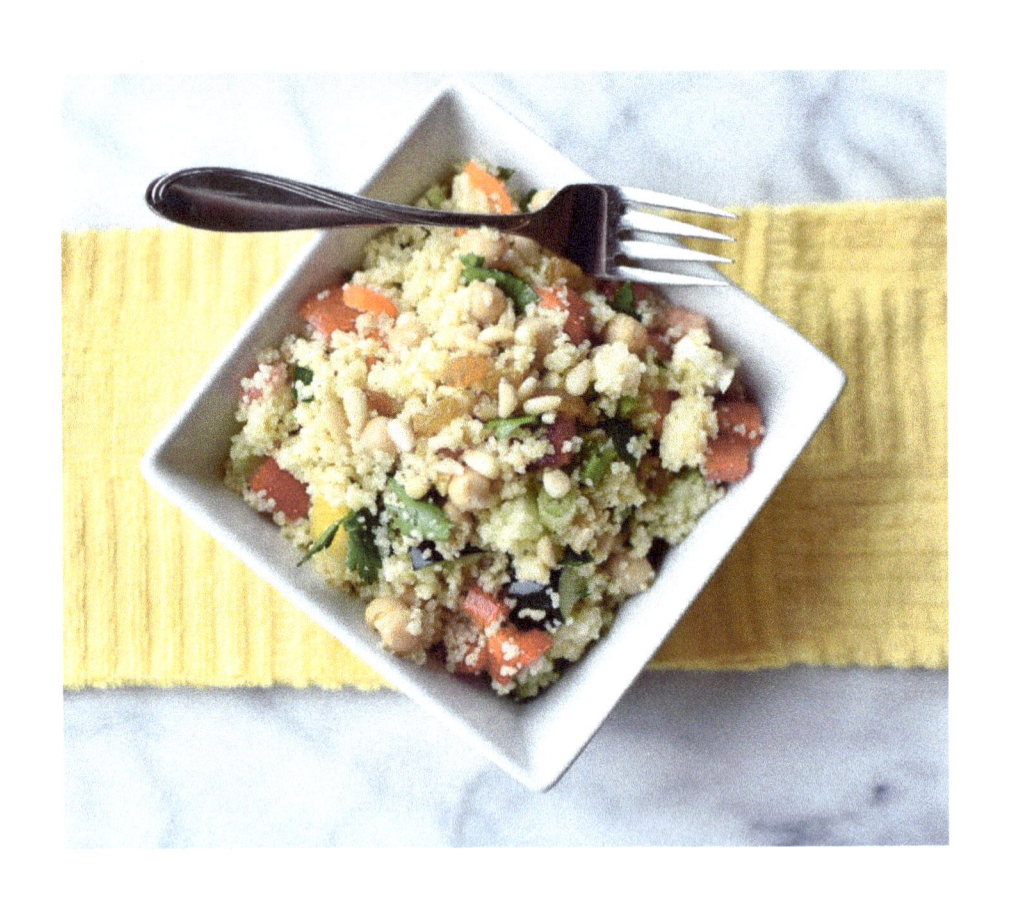

Anti-Inflammatory Blueberry Smoothie

Preparation Time: 5 minutes
Cooking Time: 5 minutes
Servings: 1

Ingredients:

1 cup Almond milk
1 Frozen banana
2/3-1 cup Frozen blueberries
2 handfuls Leafy greens/spinach
1tbsp Almond butter
25 tsp Cinnamon
Cayenne pepper
Optional: Maca powder (1 tsp.)

Directions:

1.Combine each of the fixings using a high-powered blender.

2.Mix thoroughly until creamy and serve in a chilled glass.

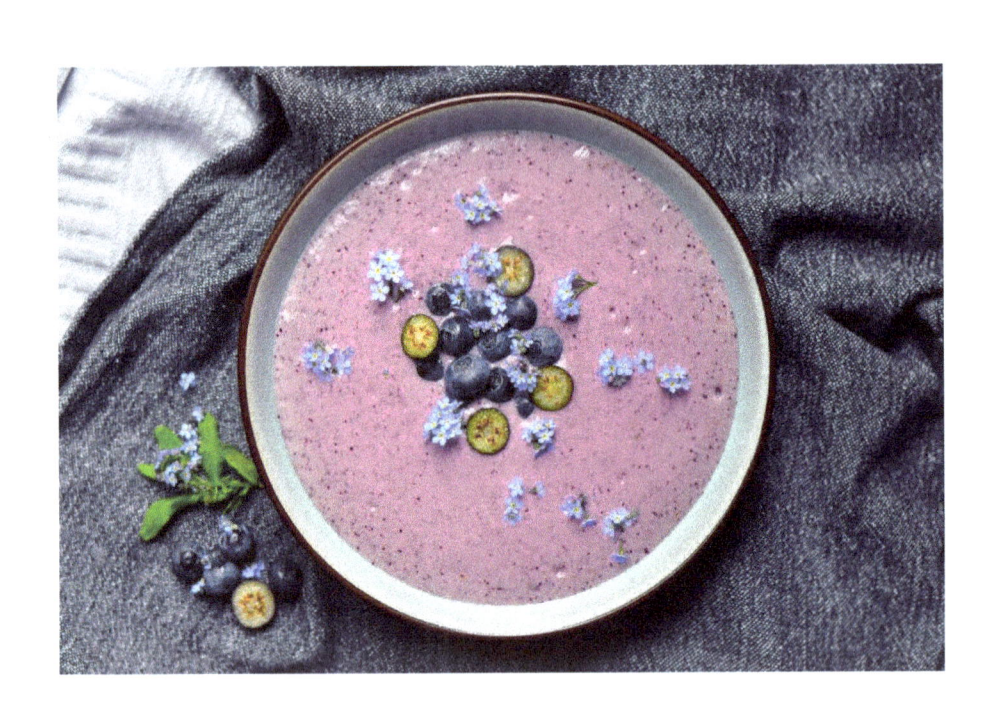

Cherry - Pomegranate Smoothie Bow - Gluten-Free & Vegetarian

Preparation Time: 5 minutes

Cooking Time: 5 minutes

Servings: 4

Ingredients:

16 oz. bag Frozen dark sweet cherries
1.5 cup 2% Plain Greek yogurt
75 cup Pomegranate juice
33 cup more as needed 2% milk
75 tsp Ground cinnamon
5 cup Fresh pomegranate seeds
5 cup Chopped pistachios
6 Ice cubes

Directions:

1. Chop the pistachios or purchase (arils) found in the produce section of the market. If you are using the whole fruit, remove the seeds underwater in a container to float to the top.

2. Add the fixings into a blender (ice, milk, cinnamon, vanilla, juice, yogurt, and cherries).

3. Pulse until it's creamy smooth. Use a little extra milk to thin the texture to get it to the desired consistency.

4.Pour the prepared smoothie into for dishes and top with two tbsp. of the chopped pistachios and two tbsp. of the seeds. Serve it immediately.

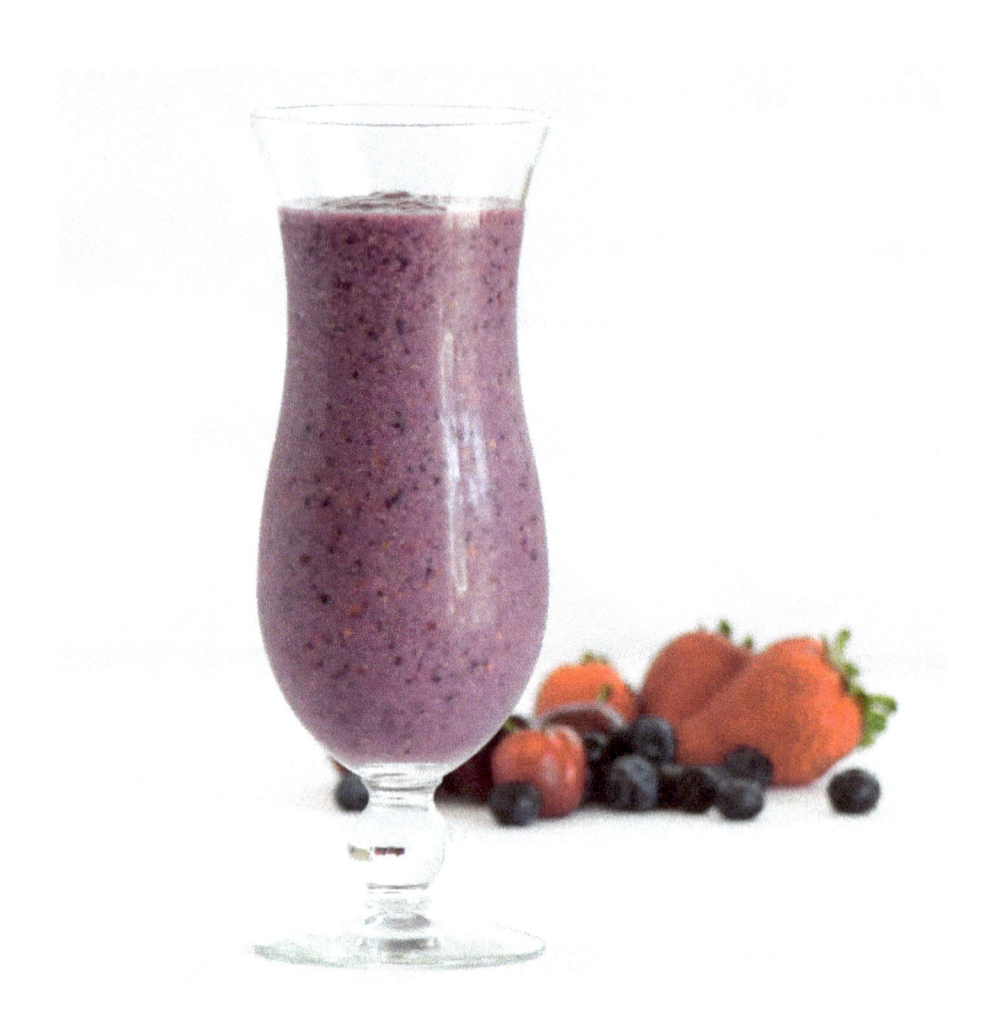

Breakfast Banana Green Smoothie

Preparation Time: 5 minutes
Cooking Time: 5 minutes
Servings: 1

Ingredients:
2 cups baby spinach leaves or 1 banana
¾ cup plain Fat-free Greek yogurt, or to taste
¾ cup ice
2 tbsp. honey
1 carrot

Directions:

1. Put spinach, banana, carrot, yogurt, ice, and honey in a blender; blend until smooth.

2. Enjoy!

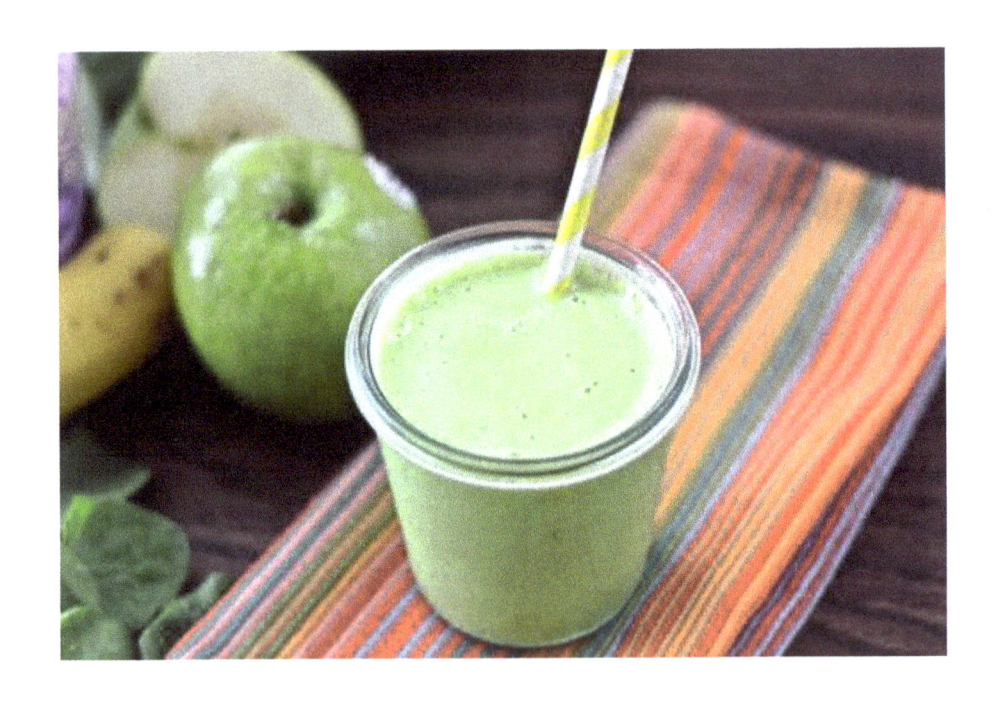

Strawberry Oatmeal Breakfast Smoothie

Preparation Time: 5 minutes
Cooking Time: 5 minutes
Servings: 2

Ingredients:

1 cup soy milk
½ cup rolled oats
1 banana, broken into chunks 14 frozen strawberries
½ tsp. vanilla extract 1 ½ tsp. white sugar

Directions:

1.In a blender, combine soy milk, oats, banana and strawberries. Add vanilla and sugar if desired. Blend until smooth.

2.Pour into glasses and serve.

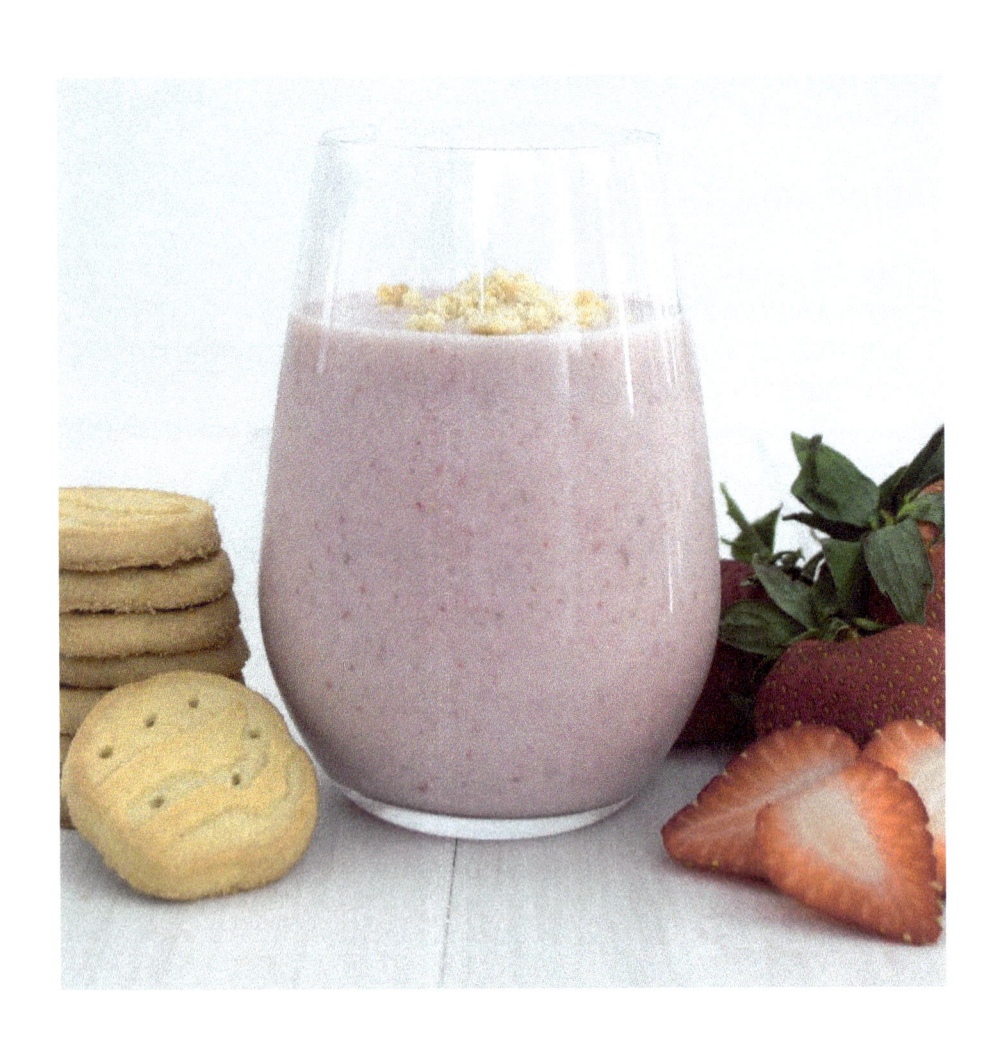

Kale and Banana Smoothie

Preparation Time: 5 minutes
Cooking Time: 5 minutes
Servings: 1

Ingredients:

1 banana
2 cups chopped kale
½ cup light unsweetened soy milk 1 tbsp. flax seeds
1 tsp. maple syrup

Directions:

1.Place the banana, kale, soy milk, flax seeds, and maple syrup into a blender. Cover, and puree until smooth. Serve over ice.

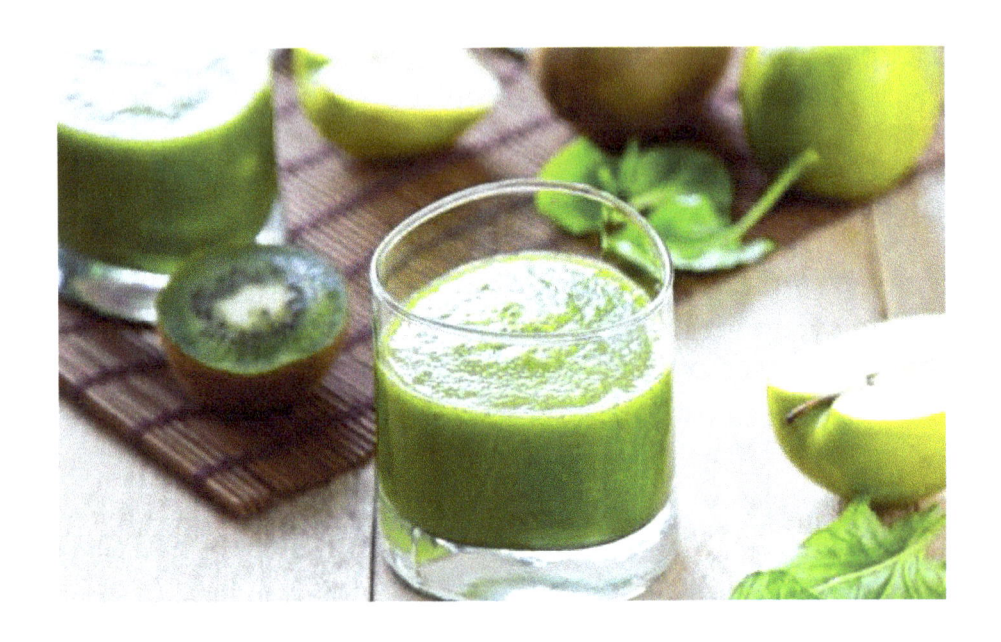

Pumpkin Pie Fall Smoothie

Preparation Time: 5 minutes
Cooking Time: 0 minutes
Servings: 3

Ingredients:

1 cup almond milk 1 tsp. agave syrup
1 cup pumpkin puree 2 tsp. cinnamon
1 apple, cored Dried cranberries

Directions:

1. Combine all ingredients except cranberries in blender and blend until smooth.

2. Top with cranberries and enjoy.

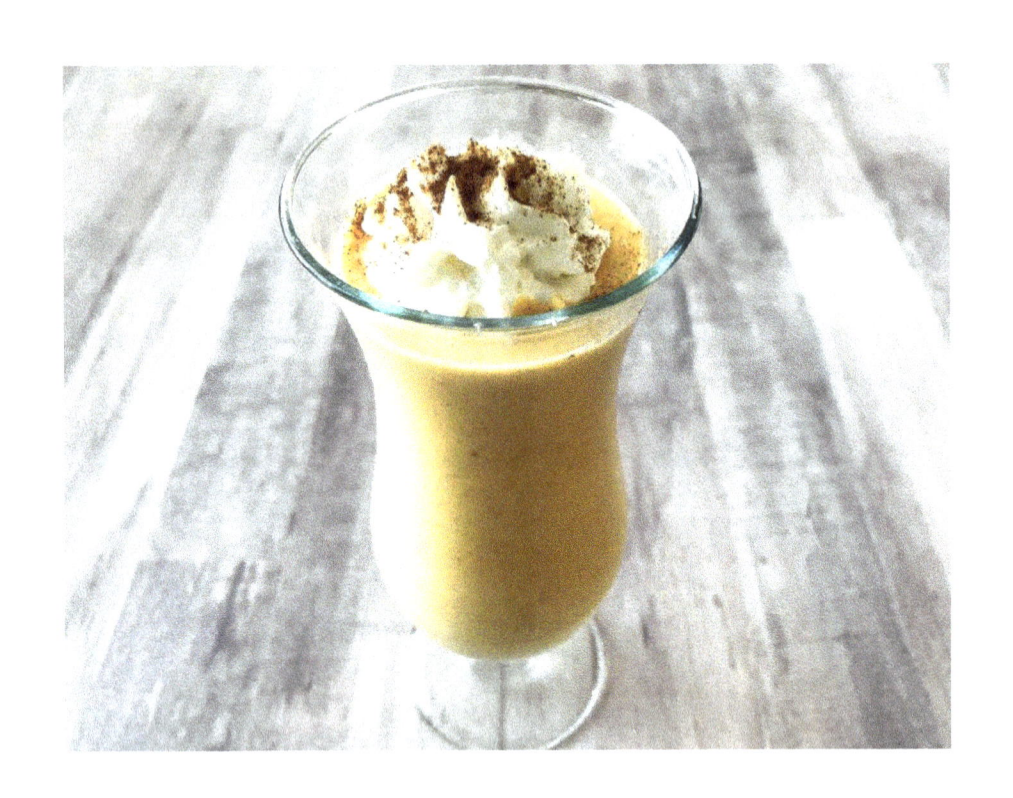

Green Tart Smoothie

Preparation Time:5 minutes

Cooking Time: 5 minutes

Servings: 1

Ingredients:

2 cups fresh kale
1 cup water
2 large stalks of celery, chopped
½ cucumber, chopped 1/3 grapefruit
1 cup frozen pineapple

Directions:

1. Blend kale and water until smooth.

2. Add remaining ingredients, and blend until smooth.

3. Enjoy!

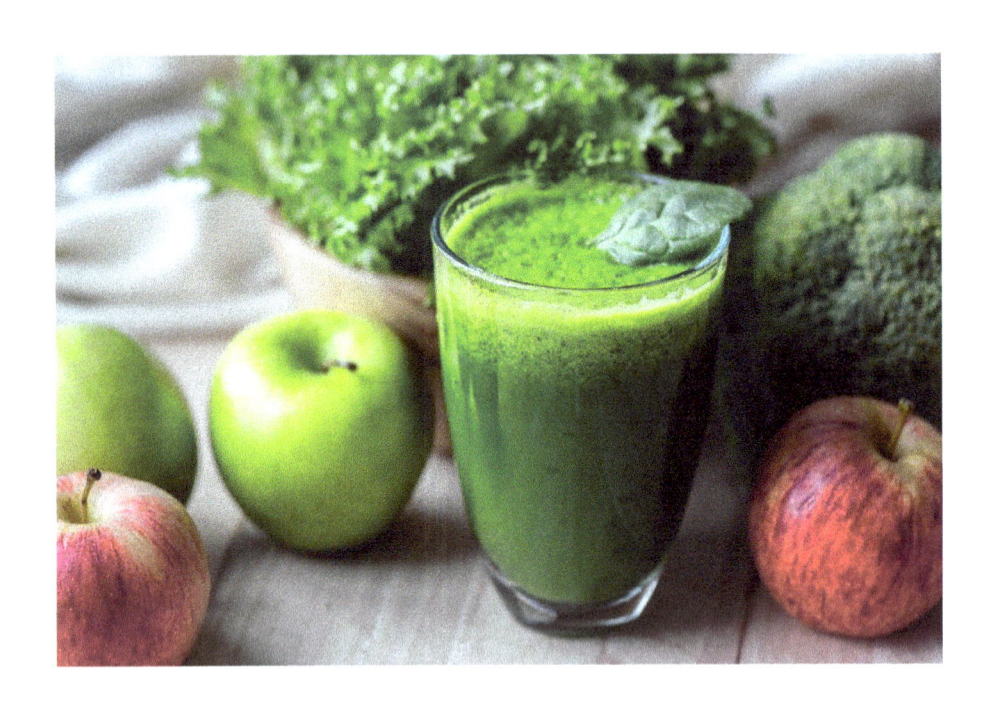

Gluten-Free Pancakes

Preparation Time: 5 minutes
Cooking Time: 2 minutes
Servings: 2

Ingredients:

6 eggs
1 cup low-fat cream cheese
1 1/12; teaspoons baking powder 1 scoop protein powder
1/4 cup almond meal 1/4 teaspoon salt

Directions:

1. Combine dry ingredients in a food processor. Add the eggs one after another and then the cream cheese. Mix it well.

2. Lightly grease a skillet with cooking spray and place over medium- high heat.

3. Pour the batter into the pan. Turn the pan gently to create round pancakes.

4. Cook for about 2 minutes on each side.

5. Serve pancakes with your favorite topping.

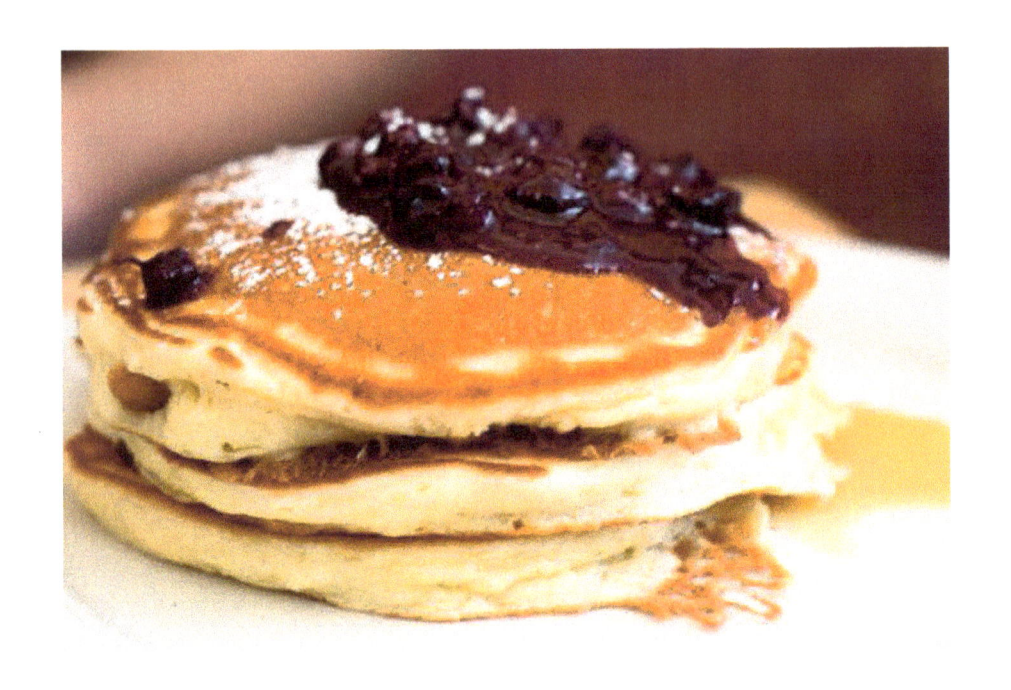

Crunchy Quinoa Meal

Preparation Time: 5 minutes
Cooking time: 25 minutes
Servings: 2

Ingredients:

3 cups coconut milk 1 cup rinsed quinoa
1/8 tsp. ground cinnamon 1 cup raspberry
1/2 cup chopped coconuts

Directions:

1. In a saucepan, pour milk and bring to a boil over moderate heat.

2. Add the quinoa to the milk and then bring it to a boil once more.

3. You then let it simmer for at least 15 minutes on medium heat until the milk is reduced.

4. Stir in the cinnamon then mix properly.

5. Cover it then cook for 8 minutes until the milk is completely absorbed.

6. Add the raspberry and cook the meal for 30 seconds.

7. Serve and enjoy.

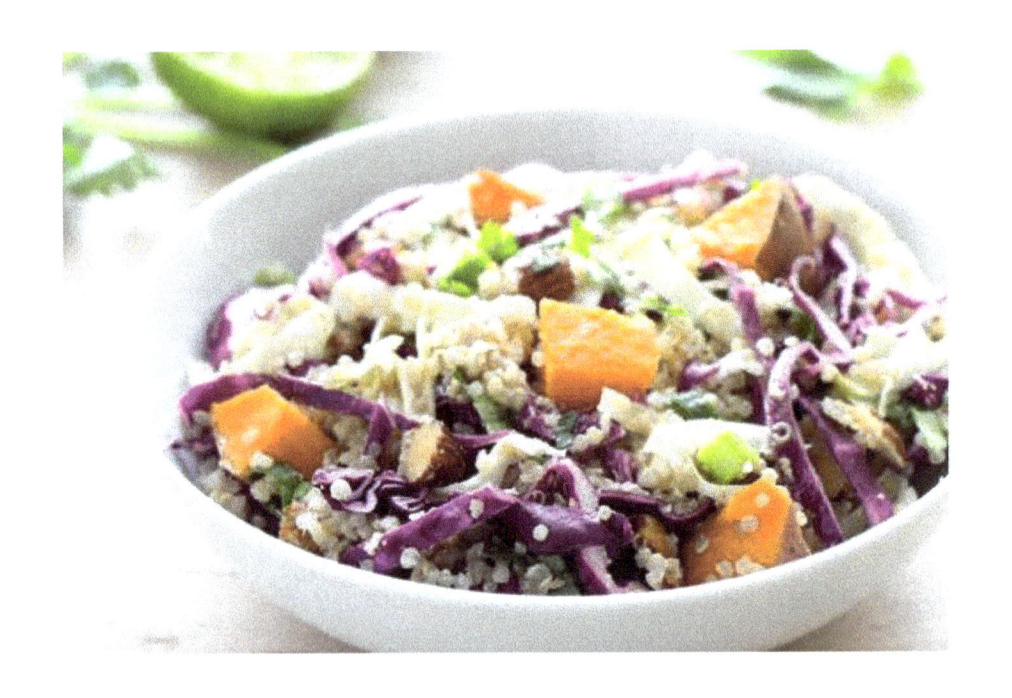

Coconut Pancakes

Preparation Time: 5 minutes
Cooking Time: 15 minutes
Servings: 4

Ingredients:

1 cup coconut flour
2 tbsps. arrowroot powder 1 tsp. baking powder
1 cup coconut milk 3 tbsps. coconut oil

Directions:

1.In a medium container, mix in all the dry ingredients.
2.Add the coconut milk and 2 tbsps. of the coconut oil then mix properly.
3.In a skillet, let melt 1 tsp. of coconut oil.

4.Pour a ladle of the batter into the skillet then swirl the pan to spread the batter evenly into a smooth pancake.

5.Cook it for like 3 minutes on medium heat until it becomes firm.

6.Turn the pancake to the other side then cook it for another 2 minutes until it turns golden brown.

7.Cook the remaining pancakes in the same process.

8.Serve.

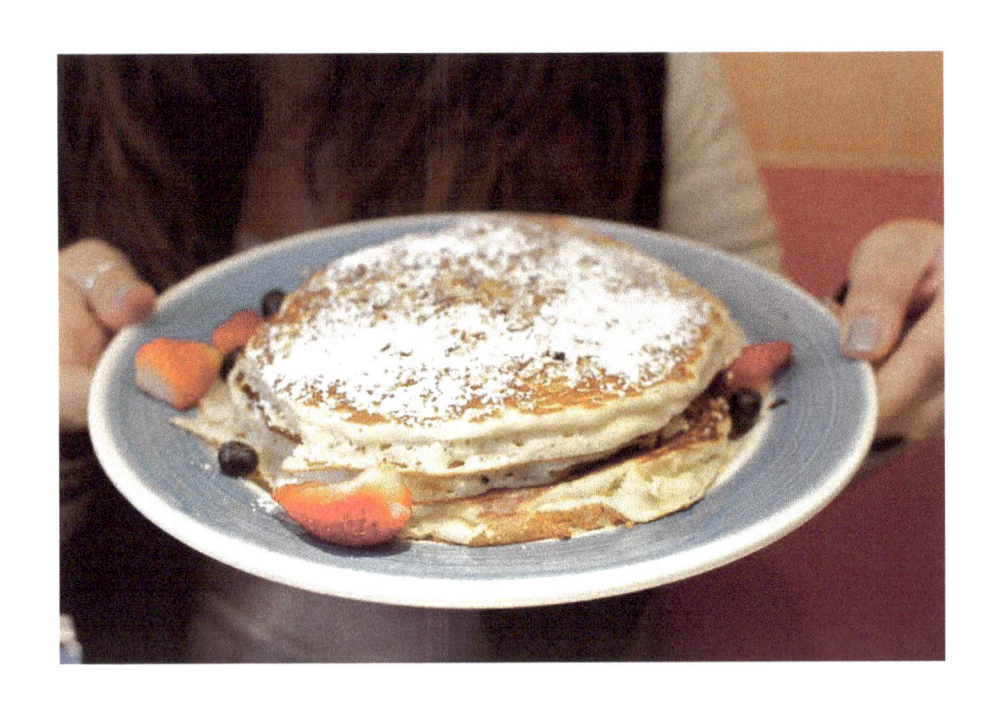

Quinoa Porridge

Preparation Time: 5 minutes
Cooking Time: 25 minutes
Servings: 2

Ingredients:

2 cups coconut milk 1 cup rinsed quinoa
1/8 tsp. ground cinnamon 1 cup fresh blueberries

Directions:

1. In a saucepan, boil the coconut milk over high heat.

2. Add the quinoa to the milk then bring the mixture to a boil.

3. You then let it simmer for 15 minutes on medium heat until the milk is reduces.

4. Add the cinnamon then mix it properly in the saucepan.

5. Cover the saucepan and cook for at least 8 minutes until milk is completely absorbed.

6. Add in the blueberries then cook for 30 more seconds.

7. Serve.

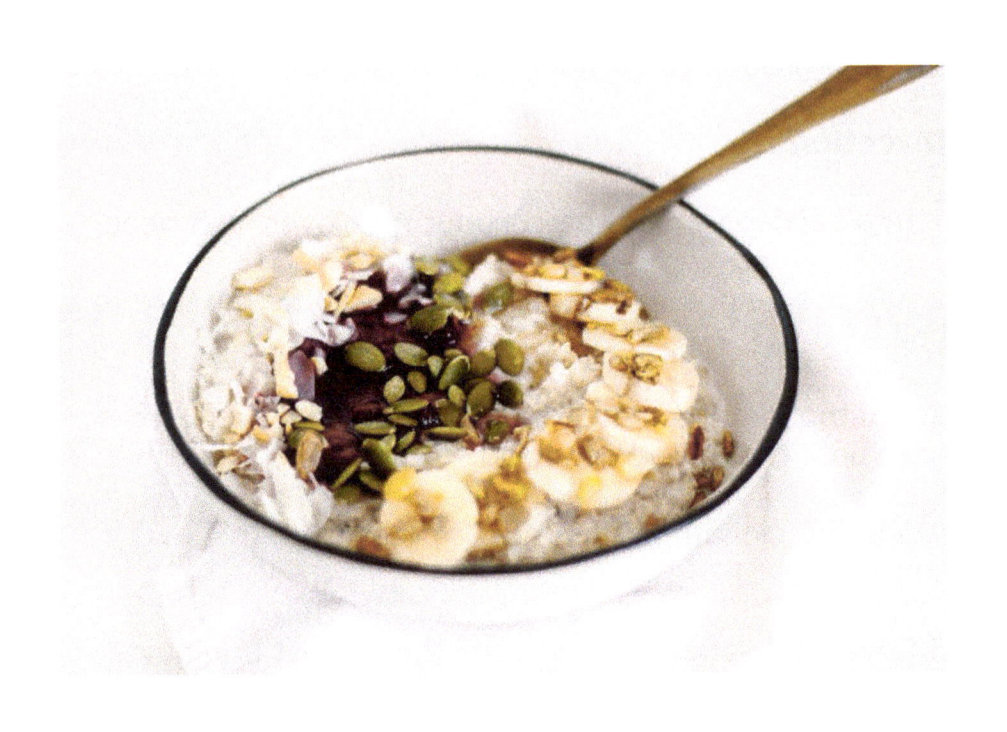

Banana barley porridge

Preparation Time: 15 minutes
Cooking Time: 5 minutes
Servings: 2

Ingredients:

1 cup divided unsweetened coconut milk 1 small peeled and sliced banana
1/2 cup barley
3 drops liquid stevia
1/4 cup chopped coconuts

Directions:

1. In a bowl, properly mix barley with half of the coconut milk and stevia.

2. Cover the mixing bowl then refrigerate for about 6 hours.

3. In a saucepan, mix the barley mixture with coconut milk.

4. Cook for about 5 minutes on moderate heat.

5. Then top it with the chopped coconuts and the banana slices.

6. Serve.

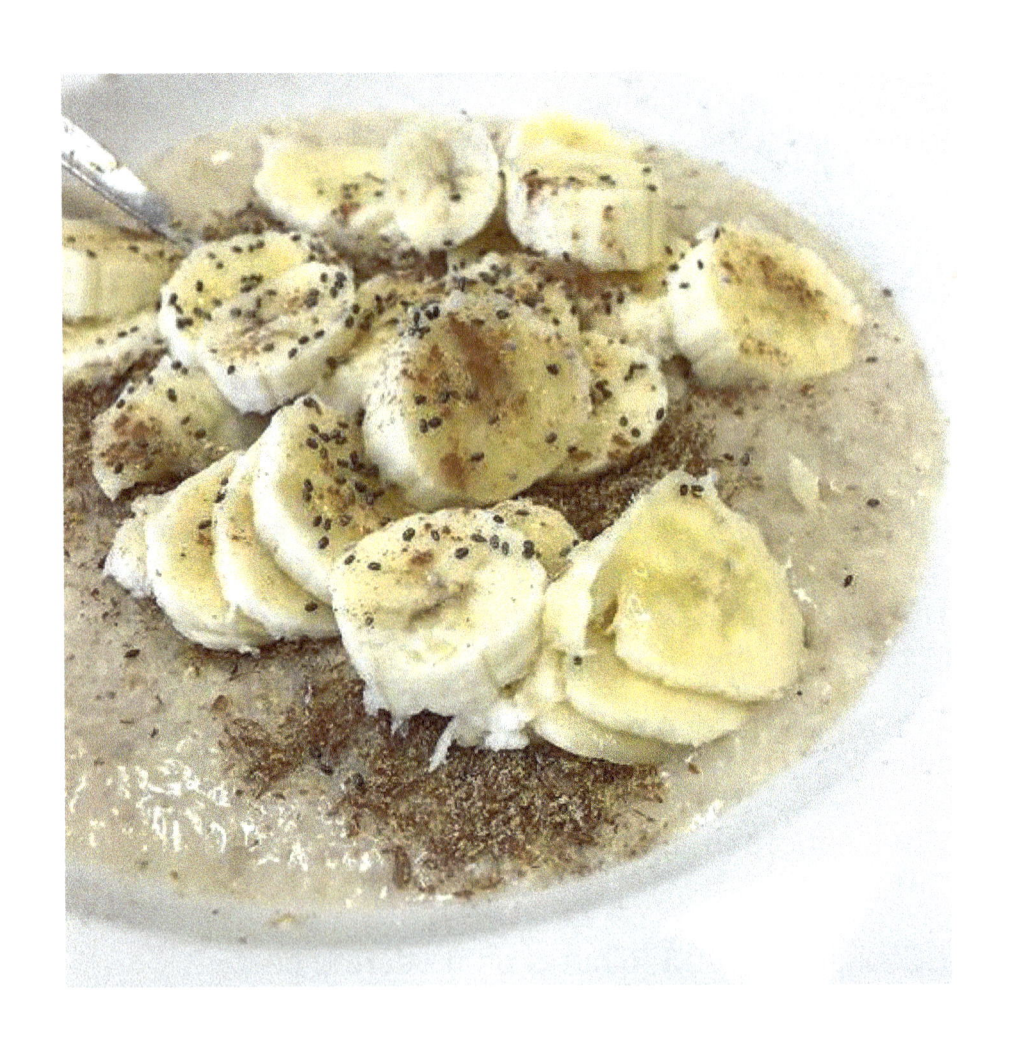

Zucchini Muffins

Preparation time: 10 minutes
Cooking time: 25 minutes
Servings: 16

Ingredients:
1 tbsp. ground flaxseed 3 tbsps. alkaline water 1/4 cup walnut butter
3 medium over-ripe bananas 2 small grated zucchinis
1/2 cup coconut milk
1 tsp. vanilla extract 2 cups coconut flour
1 tbsp. baking powder 1 tsp. cinnamon
1/4 tsp. sea salt

Directions:

1. Tune the temperature of your oven to 375ºF.

2. Grease the muffin tray with the cooking spray.

3. In a bowl, mix the flaxseed with water.

4. In a glass bowl, mash the bananas then stir in the remaining ingredients.

5. Properly mix and then divide the mixture into the muffin tray.

6. Bake it for 25 minutes.

7. Serve.

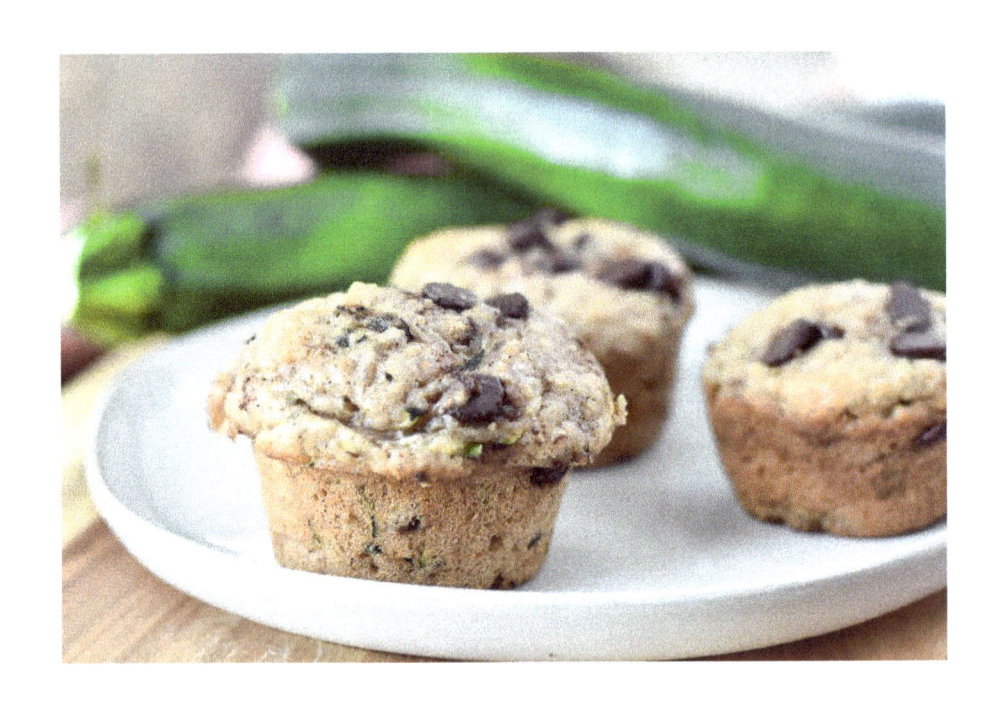

Millet Porridge

Preparation Time: 10 minutes
Cooking Time: 20 minutes
Servings:2

Ingredients:

Sea salt
1 tbsp. finely chopped coconuts 1/2 cup unsweetened coconut milk 1/2 cup rinsed and drained millet 1-1/2 cups alkaline water
3 drops liquid stevia

Directions:

1. Sauté the millet in a non-stick skillet for about 3 minutes.

2. Add salt and water then stir.

3. Let the meal boil then reduce the amount of heat.

4. Cook for 15 minutes then add the remaining ingredients. Stir.

5. Cook the meal for 4 extra minutes.

6. Serve the meal with toping of the chopped nuts.

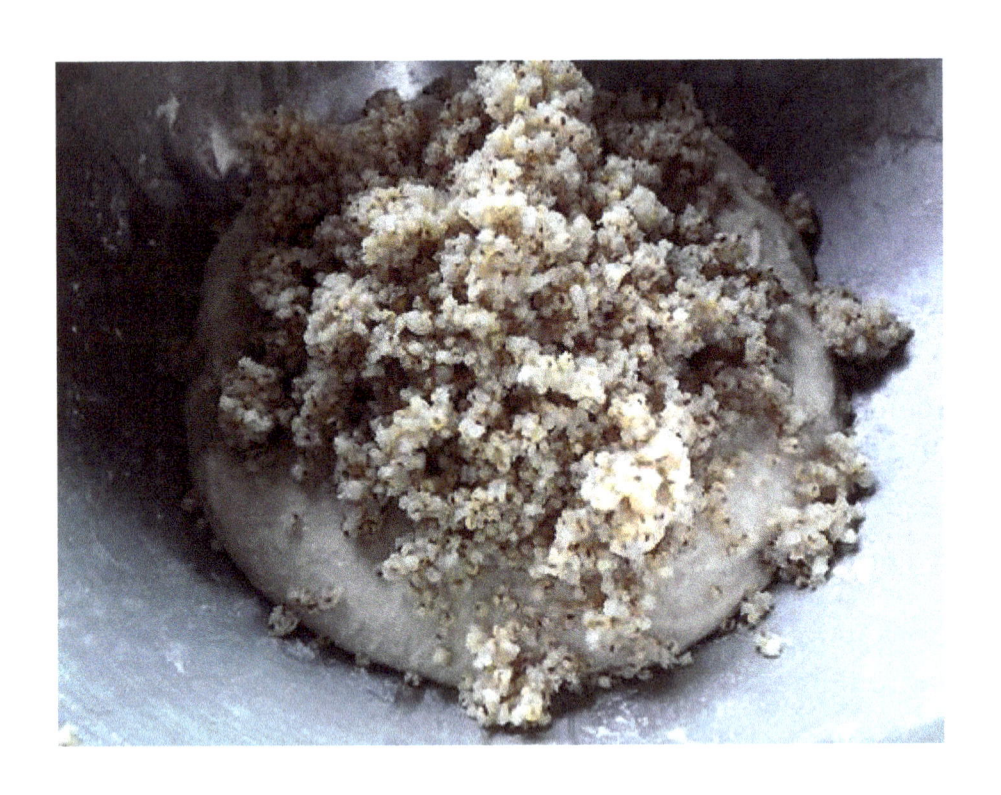

Jackfruit Vegetable Fry

Preparation Time: 5 minutes
Cooking Time: 5 minutes
Servings: 6

Ingredients:

2 finely chopped small onions
2 cups finely chopped cherry tomatoes 1/8 tsp. ground turmeric
1 tbsp. olive oil
2 seeded and chopped red bell peppers
3 cups seeded and chopped firm jackfruit 1/8 tsp. cayenne pepper
2 tbsps. chopped fresh basil leaves Salt

Directions:

1. In a greased skillet, sauté the onions and bell peppers for about 5 minutes.

2. Add the tomatoes then stir.

3. Cook for 2 minutes.

4. Then add the jackfruit, cayenne pepper, salt, and turmeric.

5. Cook for about 8 minutes.

6. Garnish the meal with basil leaves.

7. Serve warm.

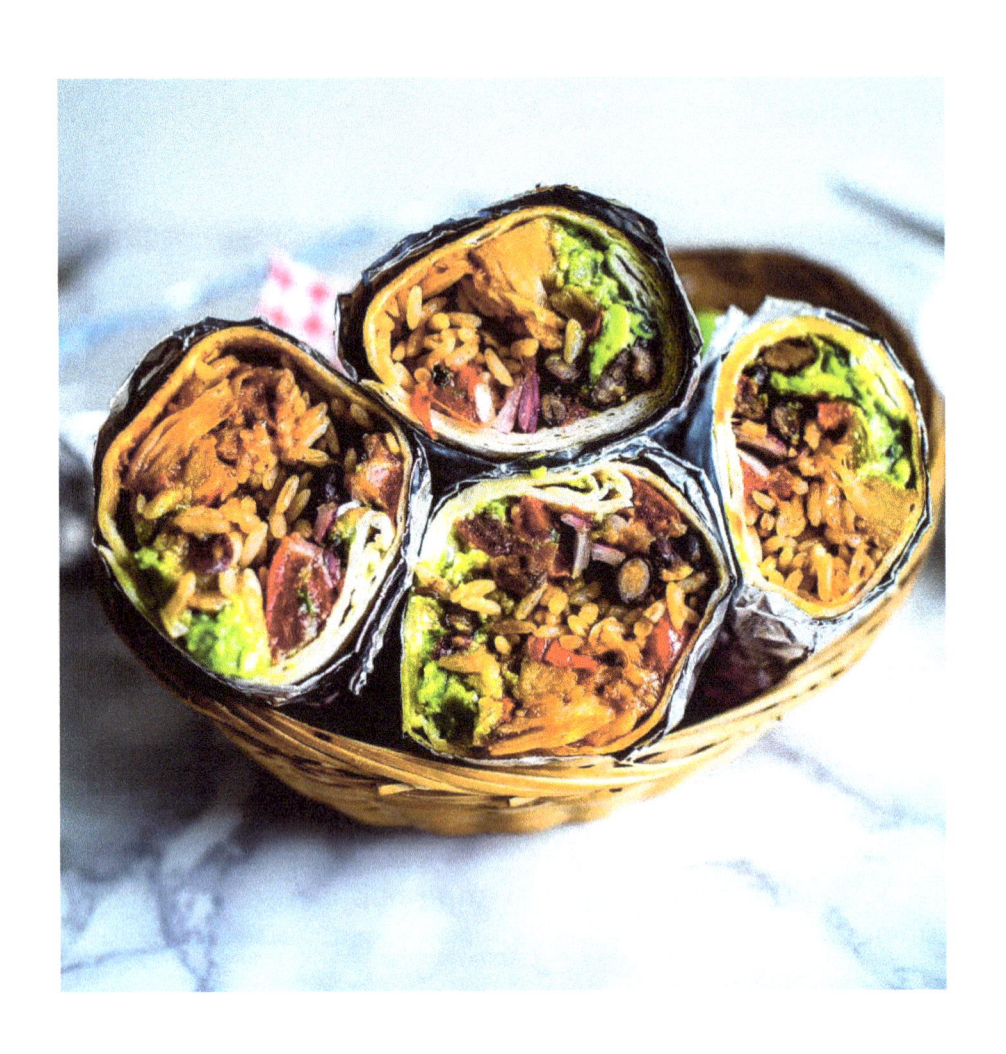

Zucchini Pancakes

Preparation Time: 15 minutes
Cooking Time: 8 minutes
Servings: 8

Ingredients:

12 tbsps. alkaline water 6 large grated zucchinis Sea salt
4 tbsps. ground Flax Seeds 2 tsps. olive oil
2 finely chopped jalapeño peppers
1/2 cup finely chopped scallions

Directions:

1. In a bowl, mix water and the flax seeds then set it aside.

2. Pour oil in a large non-stick skillet then heat it on medium heat.

3. The add the black pepper, salt, and zucchini.

4. Cook for 3 minutes then transfer the zucchini into a large bowl.

5. Add the flax seed and the scallion's mixture then properly mix it.

6. Preheat a grill then grease it lightly with the cooking spray. Pour 1/4 of the zucchini mixture into skillet then cook for 3 minutes.

7.Flip the side carefully then cook for 2 more minutes.

8.Repeat the procedure with the remaining mixture in batches.

9.Serve.

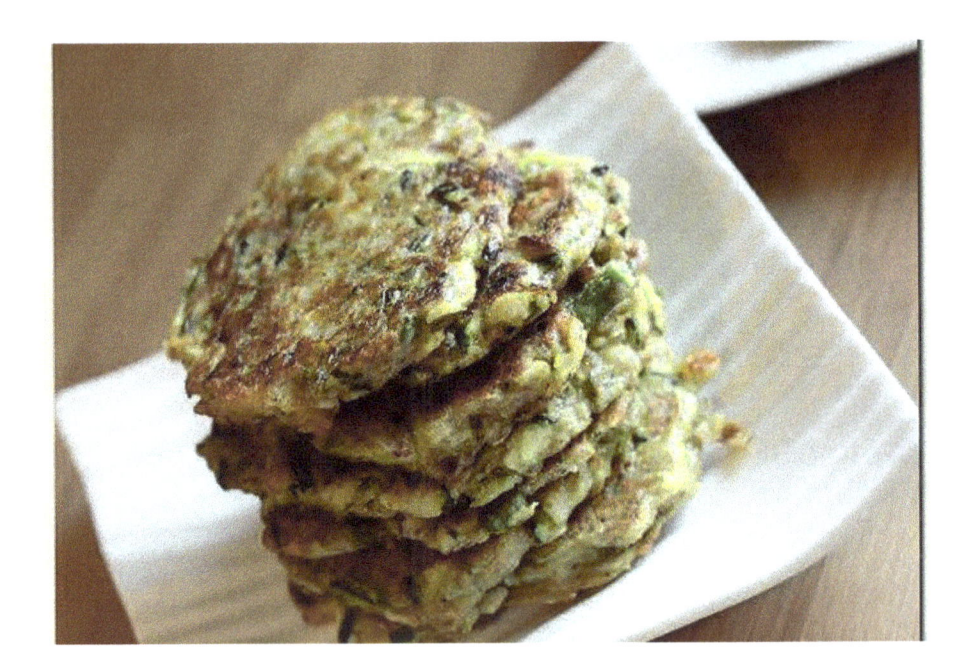

Squash Hash

Preparation Time: 2 minutes
Cooking Time: 10 minutes
Servings: 2

Ingredients:

1 tsp. onion powder
1/2 cup finely chopped onion 2 cups spaghetti squash
1/2 tsp. sea salt

Directions:

1. Using paper towels, squeeze extra moisture from spaghetti squash.

2. Place the squash into a bowl then add the salt, onion, and the onion powder.

3. Stir properly to mix them.

4. Spray a non-stick cooking skillet with cooking spray then place it over moderate heat.

5. Add the spaghetti squash to pan.

6. Cook the squash for about 5 minutes.

7. Flip the hash browns using a spatula.

8. Cook for 5 minutes until the desired crispness is reached.

9. Serve.

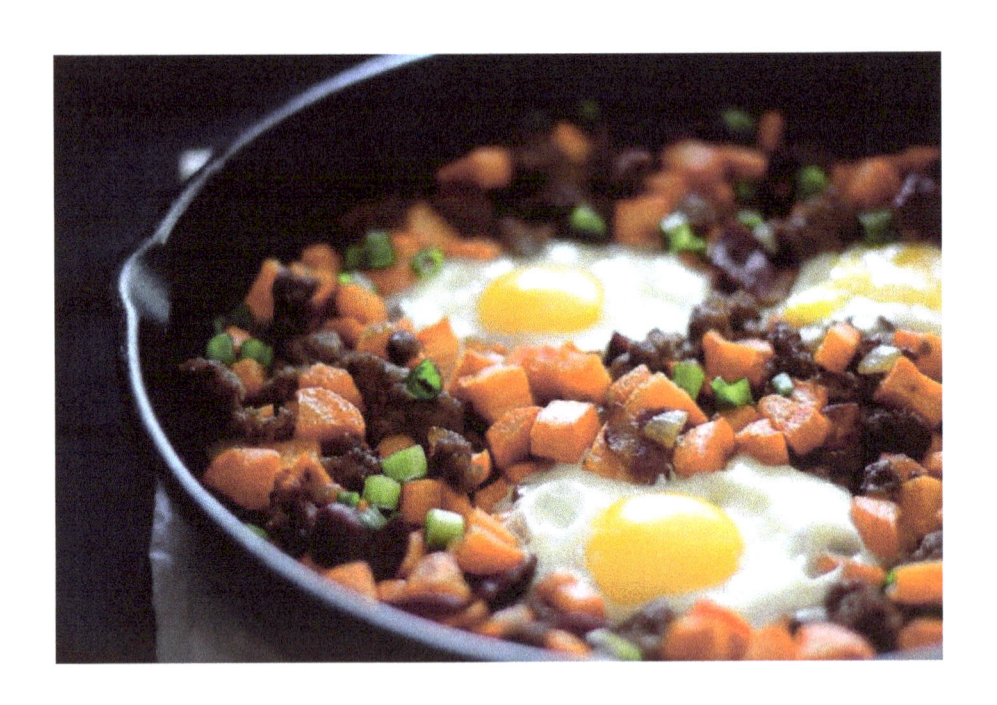

Pumpkin Spice Quinoa

Preparation Time: 10 minutes
Cooking Time: 0 minutes
Servings: 2

Ingredients:

1 cup cooked quinoa
1 cup unsweetened coconut milk 1 large mashed banana
1/4 cup pumpkin puree 1 tsp. pumpkin spice
2 tsps. chia seeds

Directions:

1. In a container, mix all the ingredients.

2. Seal the lid then shake the container properly to mix.

3. Refrigerate overnight.

4. Serve.

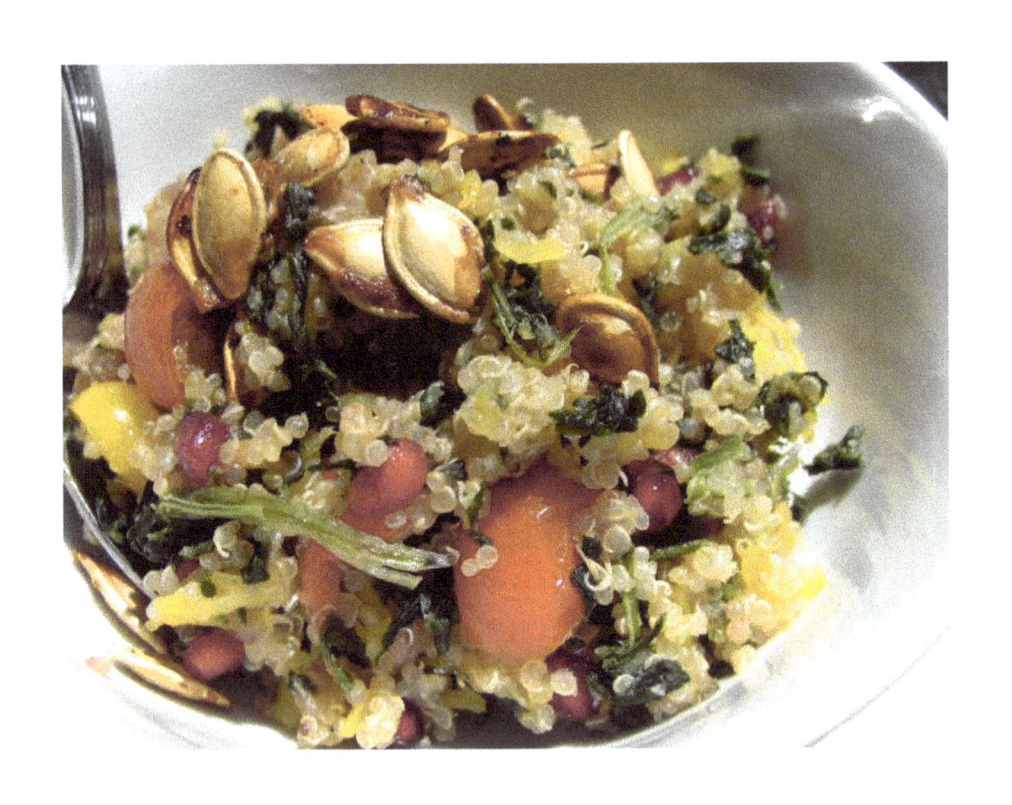

Sweet Cashew Cheese Spread

Preparation Time: 5 minutes
Cooking Time: 5 minutes
Servings: 10 servings

Ingredients:

5 drops Stevia
2 cups raw Cashews
½ cup Water

Directions:

1. Soak the cashews overnight in water.

2. Next, drain the excess water then transfer cashews to a food processor.

3. Add in the stevia and the water.

4. Process until smooth.

5. Serve chilled. Enjoy.

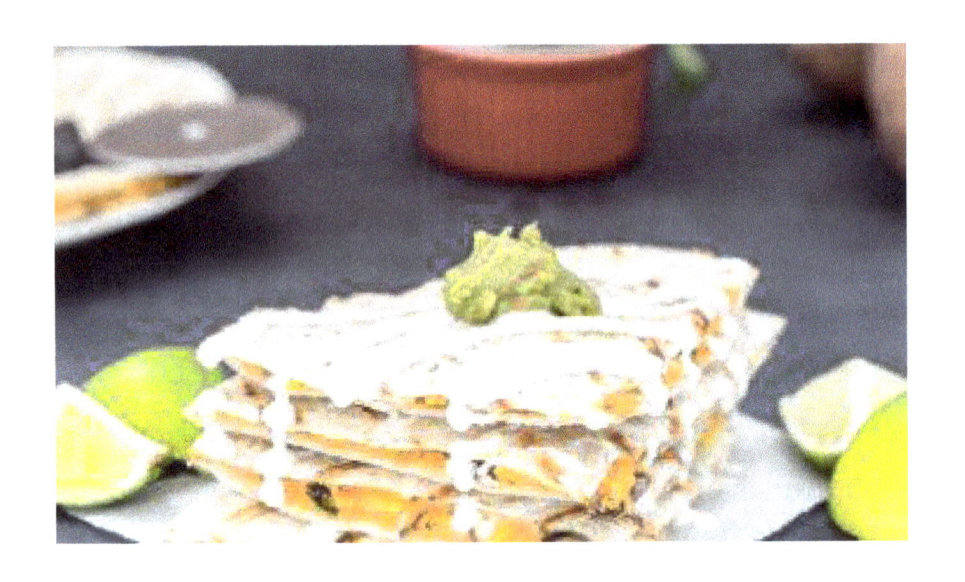

Mini Zucchini Bites

Preparation Time: 10 minutes
Cooking Time: 10 minutes
Serving**s**: 6

Ingredients:

1 zucchini, cut into thick circles 3 cherry tomatoes, halved
1 tsp. chives, chopped
1/2 cup parmesan cheese plus Salt and pepper to taste

Directions:

1. Preheat the oven to 390 degrees F.

2. Add wax paper on a baking sheet.

3. Arrange the zucchini pieces.

4. Add the cherry halves on each zucchini slice.

5. Add parmesan cheese, chives, and sprinkle with salt and pepper.

6. Bake for 10 minutes. Serve.

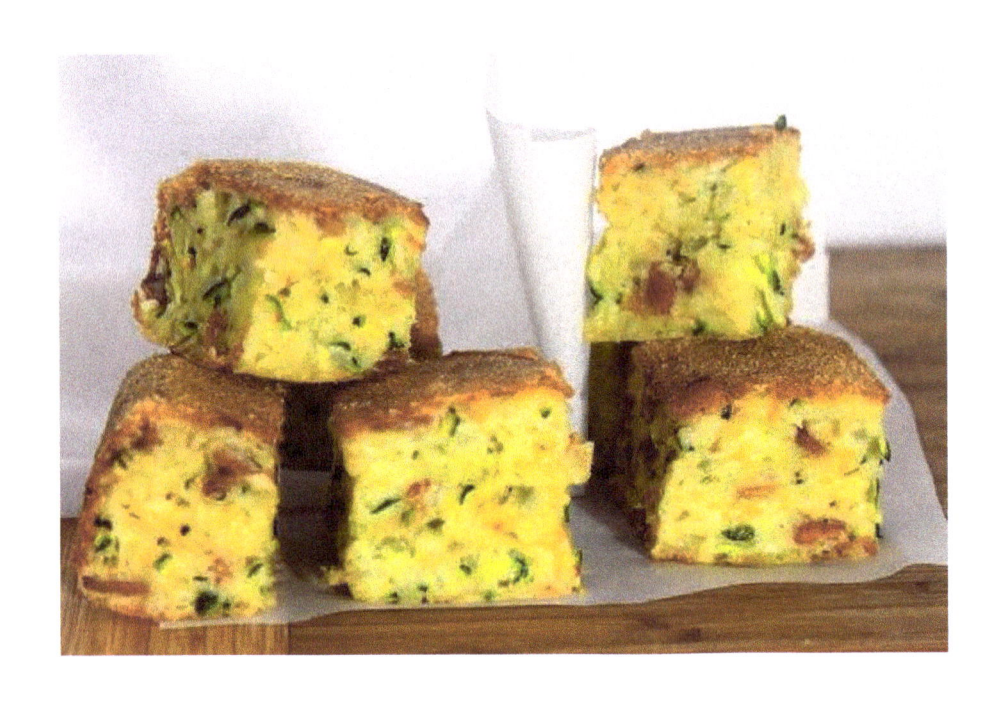

Beef with broccoli on cauliflower rice

Preparation time: 5 minutes
Cooking time: 15 minutes
Servings: 2

Ingredients:

1 lb. raw beef round steak, cut into strips.
1 Tbsp + 2 tsp low sodium soy sauce
1 Splenda packet
½ C water
1 ½ C broccoli florets
1 tsp sesame or olive oil
2 Cups cooked, grated cauliflower or frozen riced cauliflower

Directions:

1. Stir steak with soy sauce and let sit about 15 minutes.

2. Heat oil over medium-high heat then stir fry beef for 3-5 minutes or until browned.

3. Remove from pan.

4. Place broccoli, Splenda and water. Cook for 5 minutes or until broccoli start to turn tender, stirring sometimes.

5. Add beef back in and heat up thoroughly.

6. Serve the dish with cauliflower rice.

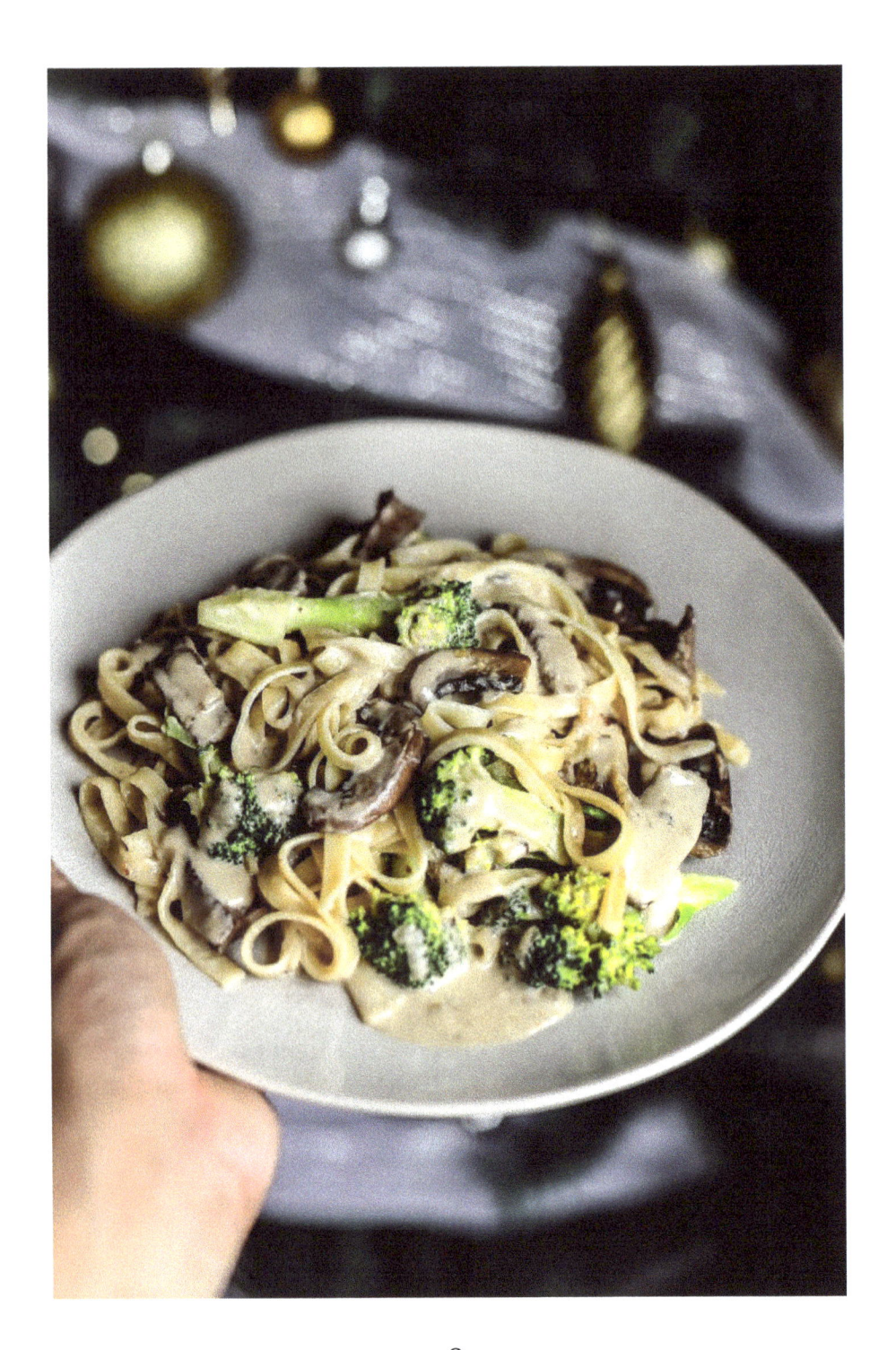

Asparagus & crabmeat frittata

Preparation time: 5 minutes
Cooking time:15 minutes
Servings: 4

Ingredients:

2½ tbsp extra virgin olive oil
plus 2 lbs. asparagus
1 tsp salt
1 ½ tsp black pepper 2 tsp sweet paprika 1 lb. lump crabmeat
1 tbsp finely cut chives
¼ cup basil chopped
4 cups liquid egg substitute

Directions:

1.Deter the tough ends of the asparagus and cut it into bite-sized pieces.

2.Preheat an oven to 375°F.

3.In a 12-Inch to a 14-inch oven-proof, non-stick skillet, warm the olive oil and sweat the asparagus until tender. Season with pepper, paprika, and salt.

4.In a mixing bowl, add the chives, crab and basil meat.

5.Pour in the liquid egg substitute and mix until combined.

6.Pour the crab and egg mixture into the skillet with the cooked asparagus and stir to combine. Bake over low to medium heat until the eggs start bubbling.

7.Place the skillet in your oven and bake for about 15-20 minutes until the eggs are golden brown. Serve the dish warm.

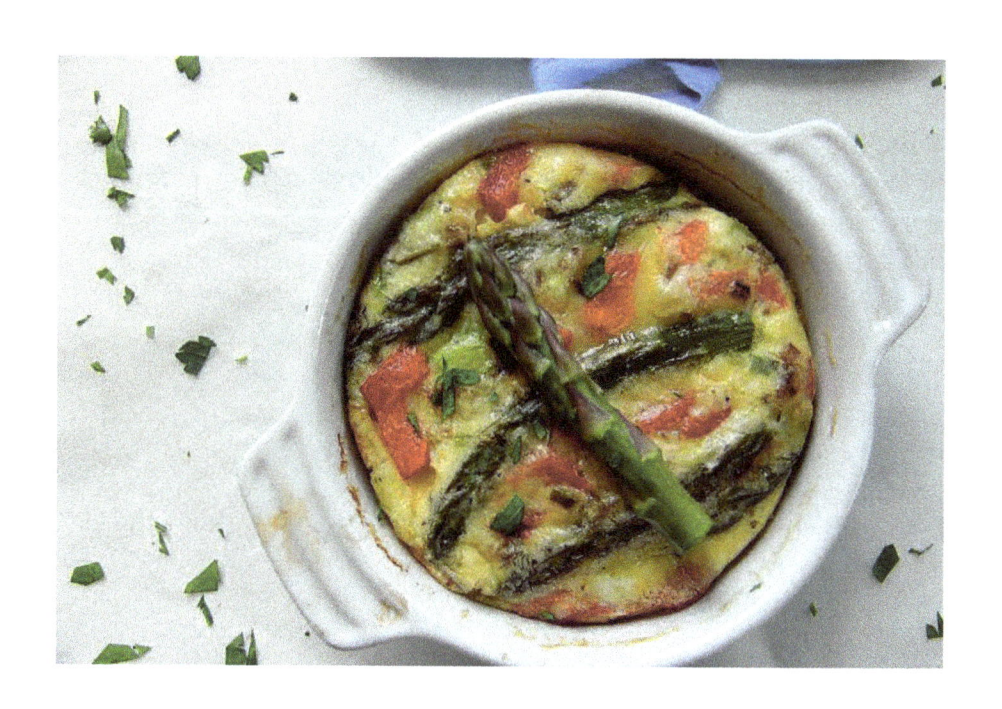

Bacon Cheeseburger

Preparation Time: 5 minutes
Cooking Time: 15 minutes
Servings: 4

Ingredients:

1 lb. lean ground beef
¼ cup chopped yellow onion and 1 clove garlic, minced
1 Tbsp. yellow mustard
1 Tbsp. Worcestershire sauce
½ tsp salt Cooking spray
4 ultra-thin slices cheddar cheese, cut into 6 equal-sized rectangular   pieces
3 pieces of turkey bacon, each cut into 8 evenly-sized rectangular pieces
24 dill pickle chips 4-6 green leaf lettuce leaves, torn into 24 small square-shaped pieces
12 cherry tomatoes, sliced in half

Directions:

1.Pre-heat oven to 400°F.

2.Combine the garlic, salt, onion, Worcestershire sauce, and beef in a medium-sized bowl, and mix well.

3.Form mixture into 24 small meatballs. Put meatballs onto a foil- lined baking sheet and cook for 12-15 minutes. Leave oven on.

4.Top every meatball with a piece of cheese, then go back to the oven until cheese melts for about 2 to 3 minutes. Let meatballs cool.

5.To assemble bites: on a toothpick layer a cheese-covered meatball, piece of bacon, piece of lettuce, pickle chip, and a tomato half.

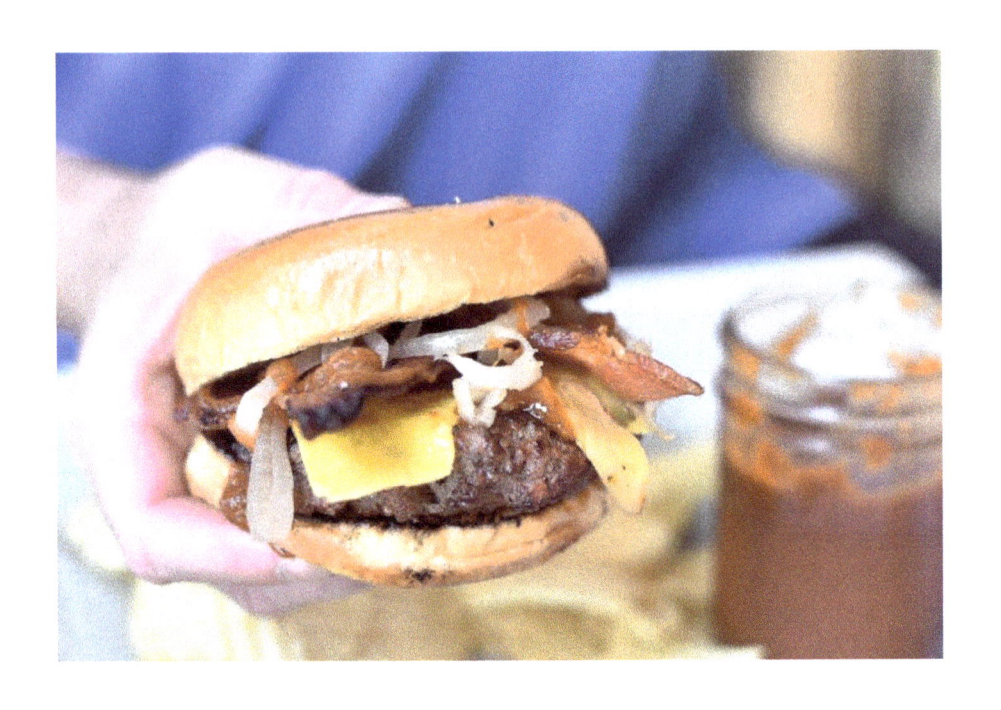

Cheeseburger pie

Preparation Time: 25 minutes
Cooking Time: 90 minutes
Servings: 4

Ingredients:

1 large spaghetti squash
1 lb. lean ground beef
¼ cup diced onion 2 eggs
1/3 cup low-fat, plain Greek yogurt 2 Tbsp. Tomato sauce
½ tsp Worcestershire sauce
2/3 cup reduced-fat, shredded cheddar cheese
2 oz dill pickle slices
Cooking spray

Directions:

1. Preheat oven to 400°F.

2. Slice spaghetti squash in half lengthwise; dismiss pulp and seeds. Spray cooking spray.

3. Place the cut pumpkin halves on a foil-lined baking sheet and bake for 30 minutes. Once cooked, let it cool before scraping the pulp from the squash with a fork to remove the spaghetti-like strings. set aside.

4. Push squash strands in the bottom and up sides of the greased pie pan, creating an even layer.

5.Meanwhile, set up pie filling. In a lightly greased, medium-sized skillet, cook beef and onion over medium heat 8 to 10 minutes, sometimes stirring, until meat is brown. Drain and remove from heat

6.The eggs, tomato paste, Greek yogurt and Worcestershire sauce and add the ground beef mixture. Pour the pie filling over the pumpkin rind.

7.Sprinkle the meat filling with cheese, then fill with pickled cucumber slices.

8.Bake for 40 minutes.

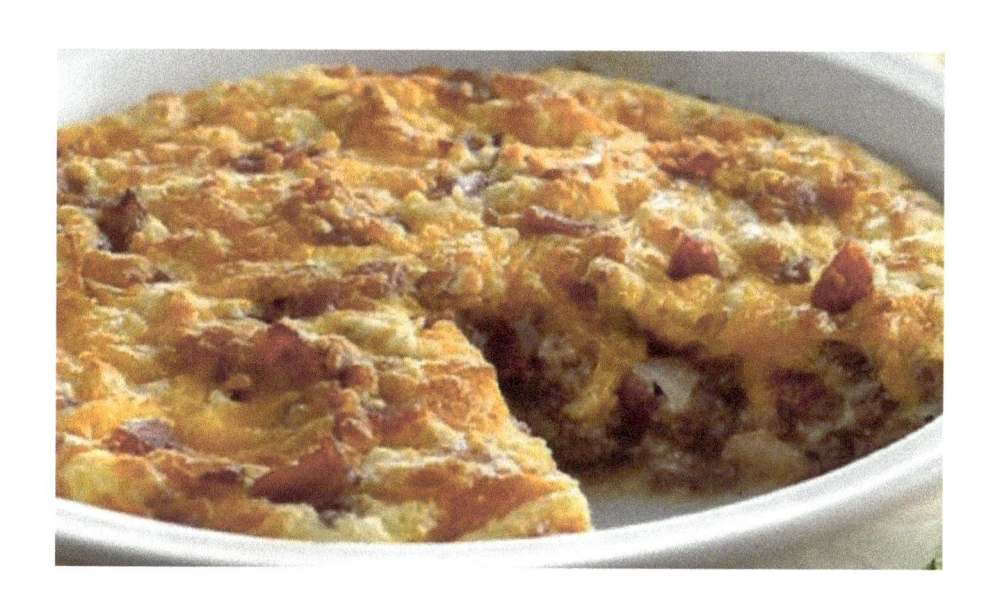

Ancho Tilapia On Cauliflower Rice

Preparation Time: 15 minutes
Cooking Time: 30 minutes
Servings: 4

Ingredients:

2 lbs. tilapia
1 tsp lime juice 1 tsp salt
1 tbsp ground ancho pepper 1 tsp ground cumin
1 ½ tbsp. extra virgin olive oil
¼ cup toasted pumpkin seeds
6 cups cauliflower rice minutes
1 cup coarsely chopped fresh cilantro

Directions:

1. Preheat oven to 450°F.

2. Dress tilapia with lime juice and set aside.

3. Combine cumin, ancho pepper, and salt in a bowl. Season tilapia with spice mixture.

4. Lay tilapia on a baking sheet or casserole dish and bake for 7 minutes.

5. In the meantime, in a big skillet, sweat the cauliflower rice in olive oil till tender, about 2-3 minutes.

6. Blend the pumpkin seeds and cilantro into the rice. Dismiss from heat, and serve.

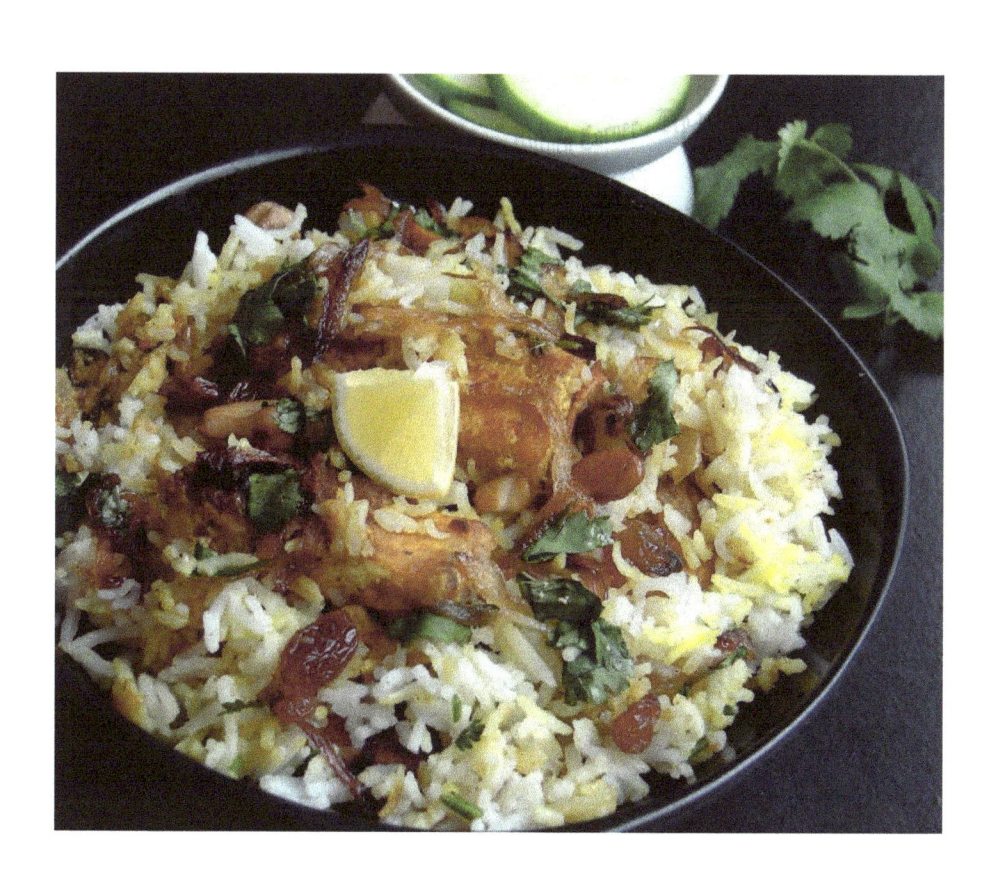

Multigrain Blueberry Yogurt Pancakes

Preparation Time: 10 minutes
Cooking Time: 20 minutes
Servings: 12-14

Ingredients:

Blueberries, one cup,
2 fresh Eggs
Salt, one-quarter teaspoon
1 cup Plain Greek yogurt
1 spoon of baking powder
1 teaspoon and one tablespoon Milk
4 tablespoons Barley or rye flour,
One-quarter of a cup All-purpose flour
One-half of a cup Butter
3 tablespoons, melted Wheat flour, one-half of a cupLemon zest,
1 teaspoon Vanilla

Directions:

1.Blend the milk, eggs, yogurt, and butter and mix the dry ingredients in another bowl.

2.Spoon the wet ingredients gently into the dry ingredients and blend.

3.Pour the batter, one-quarter of a cup for each pancake, into the hot skillet that has been oiled with a light coating of olive oil.

4. Cook each pancake for three to four minutes on each side.

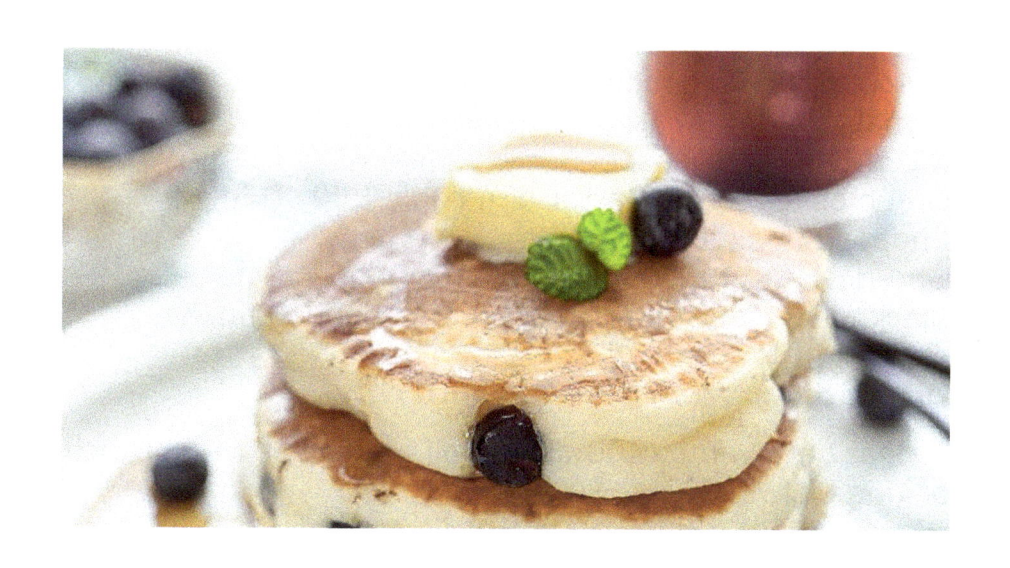

Mediterranean Frittata

Preparation Time: 5 minutes
Cooking Time: 25 minutes
Servings: 6

Ingredients:

6 eggs
Black pepper
One-quarter of a teaspoon Milk
One-quarter of a cup
Oregano, one teaspoon
Tomatoes, one-quarter of a cup
Diced Salt, one teaspoon
Green olives, one-quarter of a cup
Chopped finely Feta cheese
One-quarter of a cup, crumble
Black olives, one-quarter of a cup, chopped finely

Directions:

1.Heat the oven to 400. Spray oil an eight-by-eight-inch baking dish.

2.Beat the milk into the eggs, and then add the other ingredients.

3. Pour this mixture into the baking dish and bake for twenty minutes.

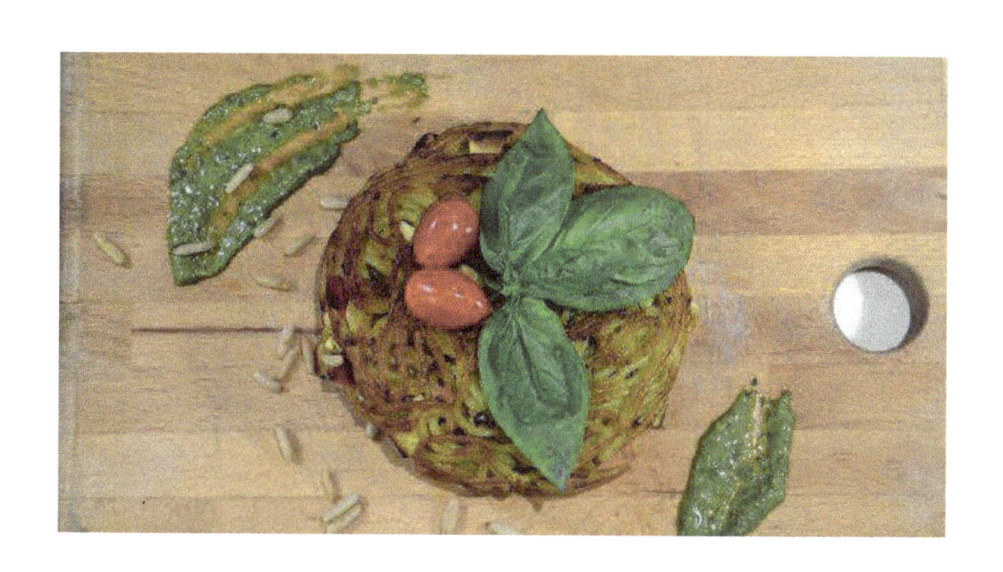

Banana Blueberry Muffins

Preparation Time: 20 minutes
Cooking Time: 25 minutes
Servings: 12

Ingredients:

Mashed ripe banana

Three-fourths of a cup Blueberries
One-half cups, fresh or frozen Milk
Three-fourths of a cupWalnuts
One-half cup, chopped finely Apple cider vinegar
One teaspoon Applesauce
One-half of a cup Baking soda
One-half of a teaspoon Vanilla
One teaspoonSea salt
One-half of a teaspoon Olive oil
One-quarter of a cup Cinnamon
One and one-half teaspoon ground Flour
Two cups Baking powder

Directions:

1.Heat the oven to 350. Spray oil in the twelve-cup muffin pan.

2.Mix the vanilla, vinegar, milk, and bananas.

3.Mix in a separate bowl the baking soda, salt, cinnamon, baking powder, and flour.

4.Mix the wet ingredients into the dry ones.

5.Fold in the blueberries and walnuts. Pour your batter into the muffin cups, and let it bake for twenty-five minutes.

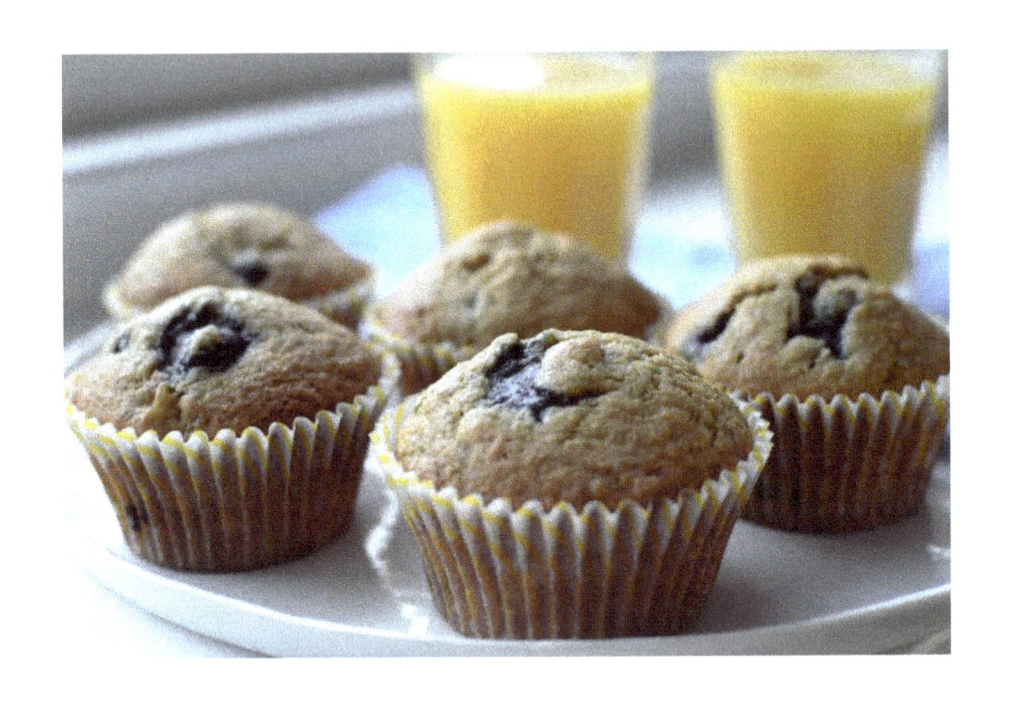

Spiced Chickpeas Bowls

Preparation time: 10 minutes
Cooking time: 30 minutes
Servings: 4

Ingredients:

15 ounces canned chickpeas, drained and rinsed
¼ teaspoon cardamom, ground
½ teaspoon cinnamon powder
1 and ½ teaspoons turmeric powder 1 teaspoon coriander, ground
1 tablespoon olive oil
A pinch of salt and black pepper
¾ cup Greek yogurt
½ cup green olives, pitted and halved
½ cup cherry tomatoes, halved 1 cucumber, sliced

Directions:

1.Spread the chickpeas on a baking sheet, add the cardamom, cinnamon, turmeric, coriander, the oil, salt and pepper, toss and bake at 375 degrees F for 30 minutes.

2.In a bowl, combine the roasted chickpeas with the rest of the ingredients, toss, and serve breakfast.

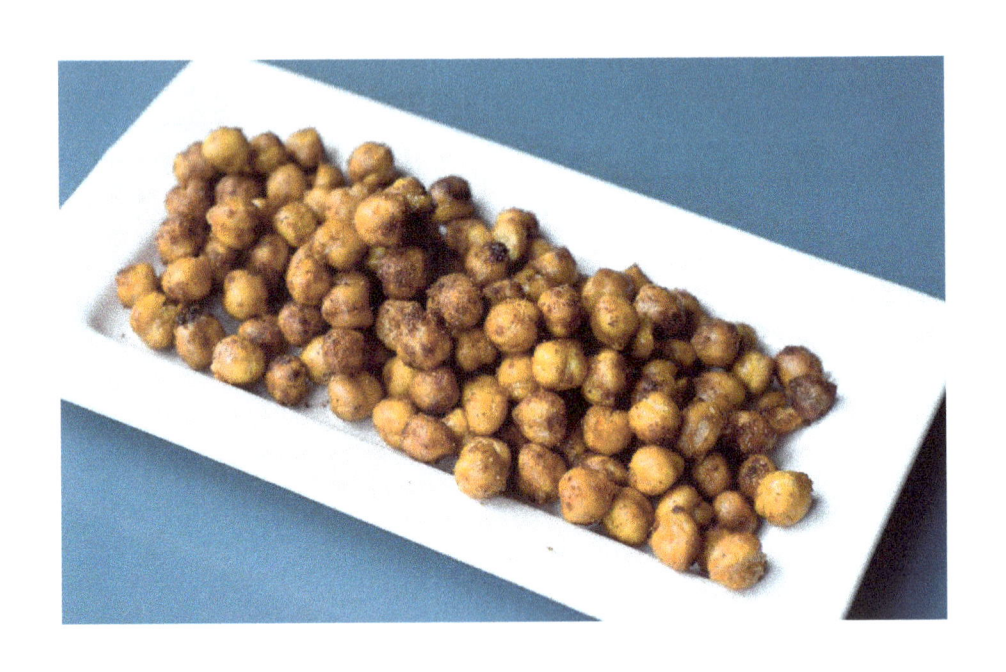

Avocado Spread

Preparation time: 5 minutes
Cooking time: 0 minutes
Servings: 8

Ingredients:

2 avocados roughly chopped
1 tablespoon sun-dried tomatoes, chopped
2 tablespoons lemon juice
3 tablespoons cherry tomatoes, chopped
¼ cup red onion, chopped 1 teaspoon oregano, dried
2 tablespoons parsley, chopped
4 kalamata olives, pitted and chopped A pinch of salt and black pepper

Directions:

1. Put your avocados into a bowl and mash with a fork.
2. Add the rest of the ingredients, stir to combine and serve as a morning spread.

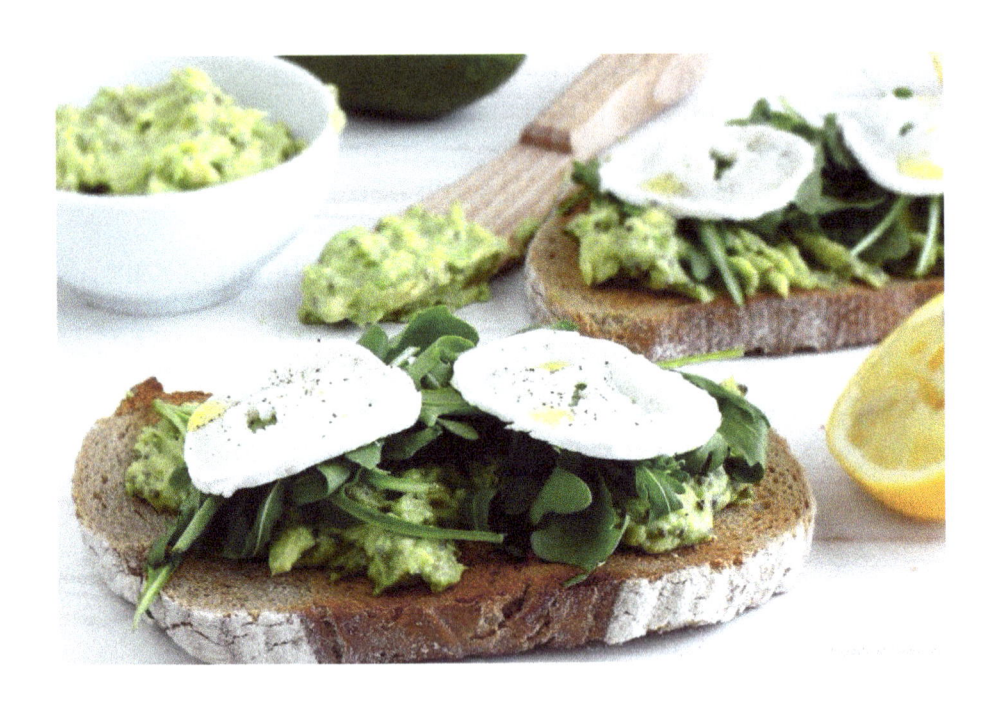

Baked Omelet Mix

Preparation time: 10 minutes
Cooking time: 45 minutes
Servings: 12

Ingredients:

12 eggs, whisked
8 ounces spinach, chopped 2 cups almond milk
12 ounces canned artichokes, chopped 2 garlic cloves, minced
5 ounces feta cheese, crumbled 1 tablespoon dill, chopped
1 teaspoon oregano, dried 1 teaspoon lemon pepper A pinch of salt
4 teaspoons olive oil

Directions:

1. Heat a pan with the oil over medium-high heat, add the garlic and the spinach and sauté for 3 minutes.

2. In a baking dish, combine the eggs with the artichokes and the rest of the ingredients.
3. Add the spinach mix and toss a bit, bake the mix at 375 degrees F for 40 minutes, divide between plates and serve for breakfast.

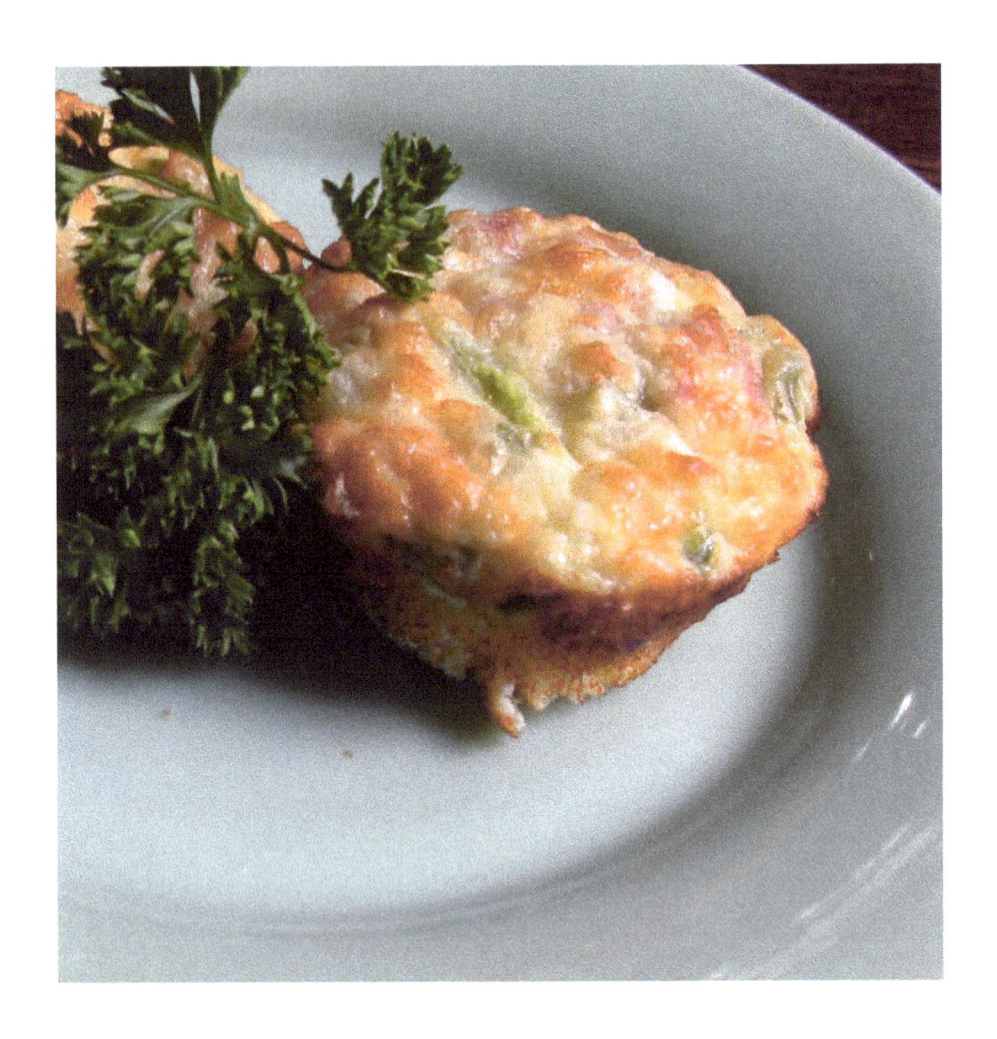

Veggie Bowls

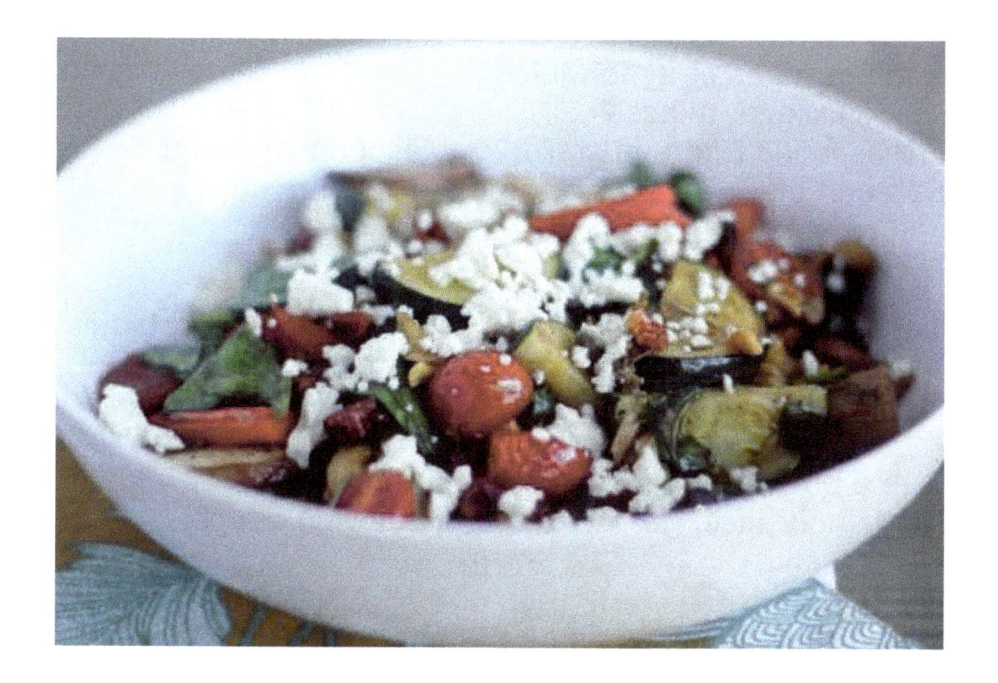

Preparation time: 10 minutes
Cooking time: 5 minutes
Servings: 4

Ingredients:

1 tablespoon olive oil
1- pound asparagus, trimmed and roughly chopped
3 cups kale, shredded
3 cups Brussels sprouts, shredded
½ cup hummus

1 avocado, peeled, pitted and sliced 4 eggs, soft boiled, peeled and sliced

For the dressing:

2 tablespoons of lemon juice
1 garlic clove, minced
2 teaspoons Dijon mustard 2 tablespoons olive oil
Salt and black pepper to the taste

Directions:

1. Heat a pan with 2 tablespoons oil over medium-high heat, add the asparagus and sauté for 5 minutes stirring often.

2. In a bowl, combine the other 2 tablespoons oil with the lemon juice, garlic, mustard, salt and pepper and whisk well.

3. In a salad bowl, combine the asparagus with the kale, sprouts, hummus, avocado and the eggs and toss gently.

4. Add the dressing, toss and serve for breakfast.

Mediterranean Egg Cups

Preparation Time: 15 minutes
Cooking Time: 25 minutes
Servings: 6

Ingredients:

On cup Bell pepper chopped finely
Feta cheese three tablespoons crumbled small
Mushrooms, one cup chopped finely
Eggs, ten
Black pepper
one-quarter of a teaspoon Milk
two-thirds of a cup
Salt
one-quarter of a teaspoon Garlic powder
one teaspoon Spray oil

Directions:

1. Heat the oven to 350. Spray oil in the twelve-muffin cup pan.

2. Add the pepper, salt, garlic powder, and milk into the beaten egg until mixed well.

3. Add in the peppers and the mushrooms. Fill the muffin pan cups with this mix.

4. Bake for twenty-five minutes.

5.Cool for five minutes then top with the cheese and serve.

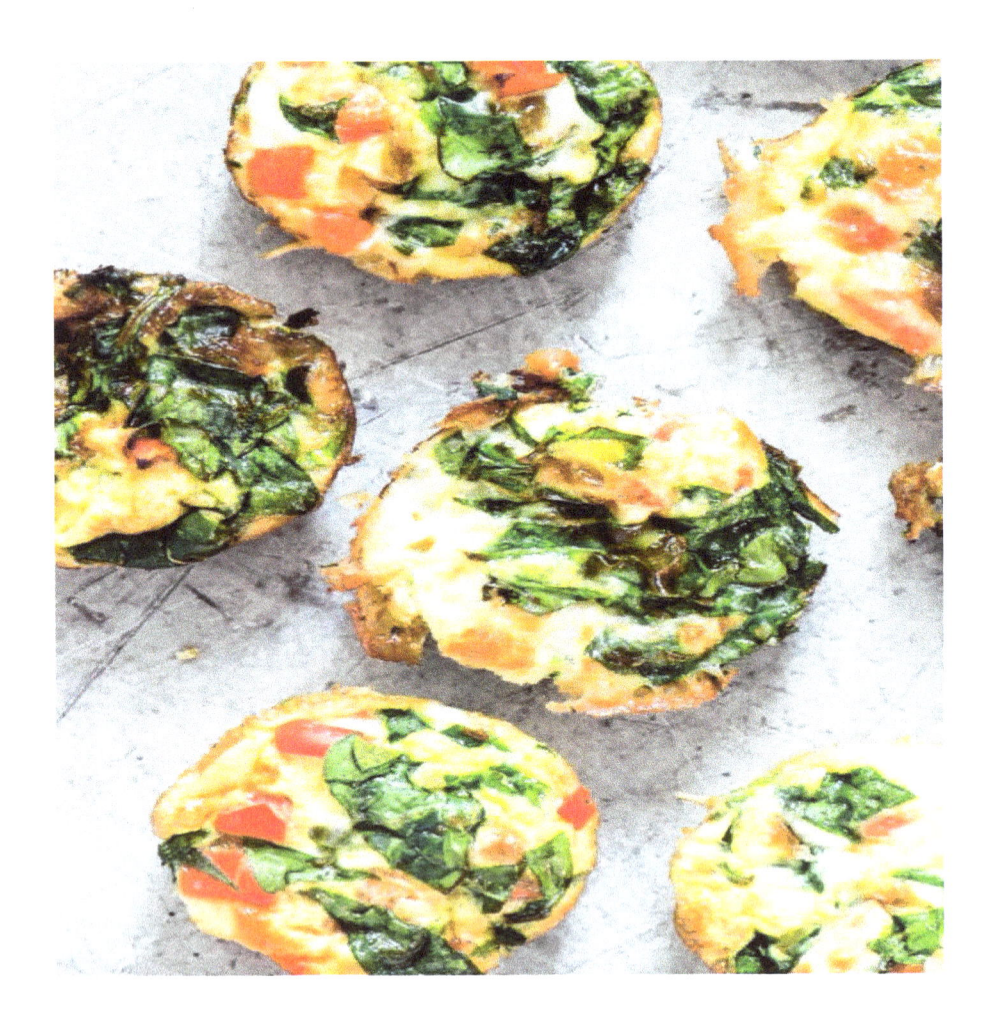

Avocado and Apple Smoothie

Preparation time: 5 minutes
Cooking time: 0 minutes
Servings: 2

Ingredients:

2 cups spinach
1 green apple, cored and chopped
1 avocado, peeled, pitted and chopped 3 tablespoons chia seeds
1 teaspoon honey
1 banana, frozen and peeled 2 cups coconut water

Directions:

1.In your blender, combine the spinach with the apple and the rest of the ingredients, pulse, divide into glasses and serve.

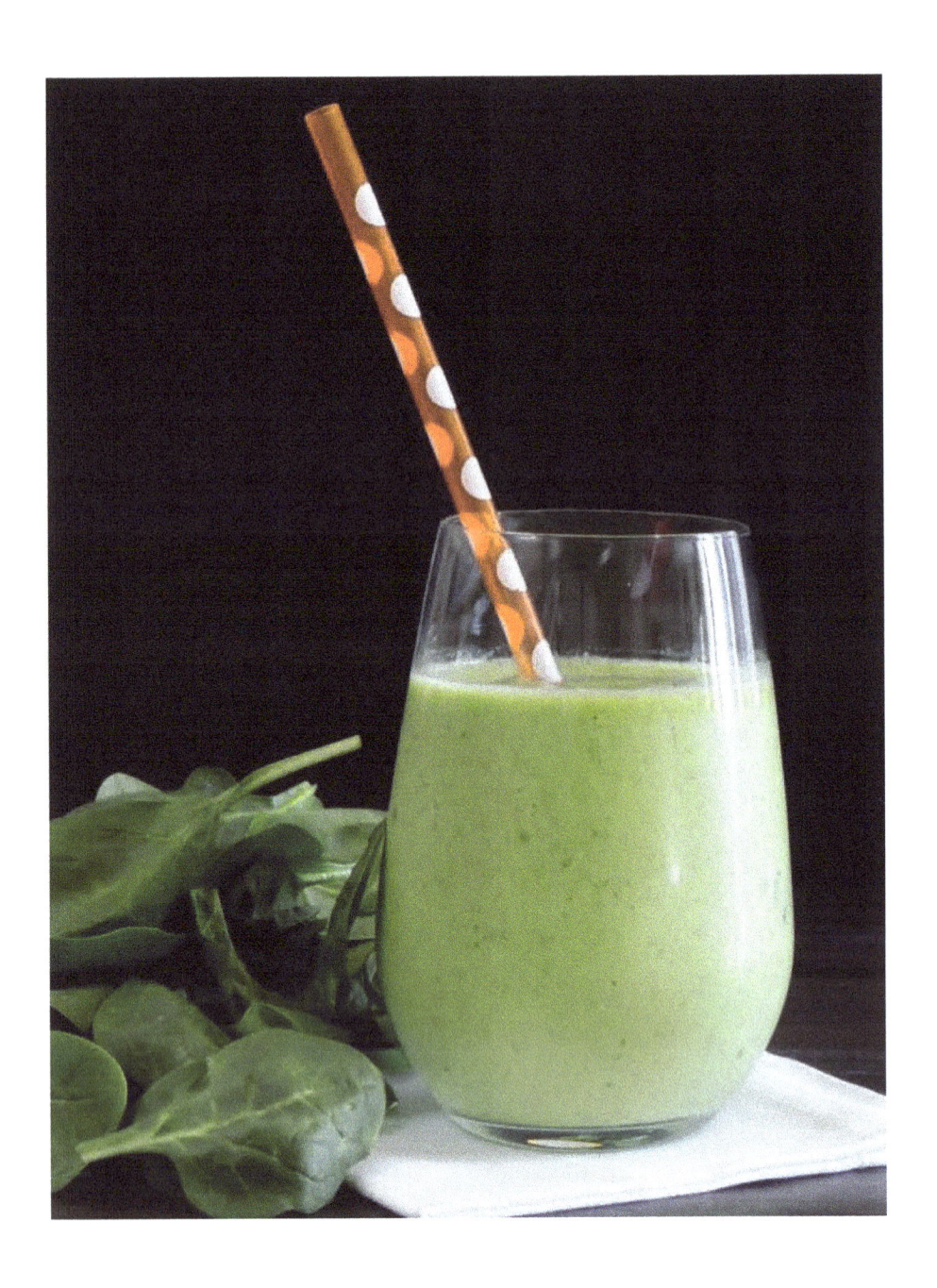

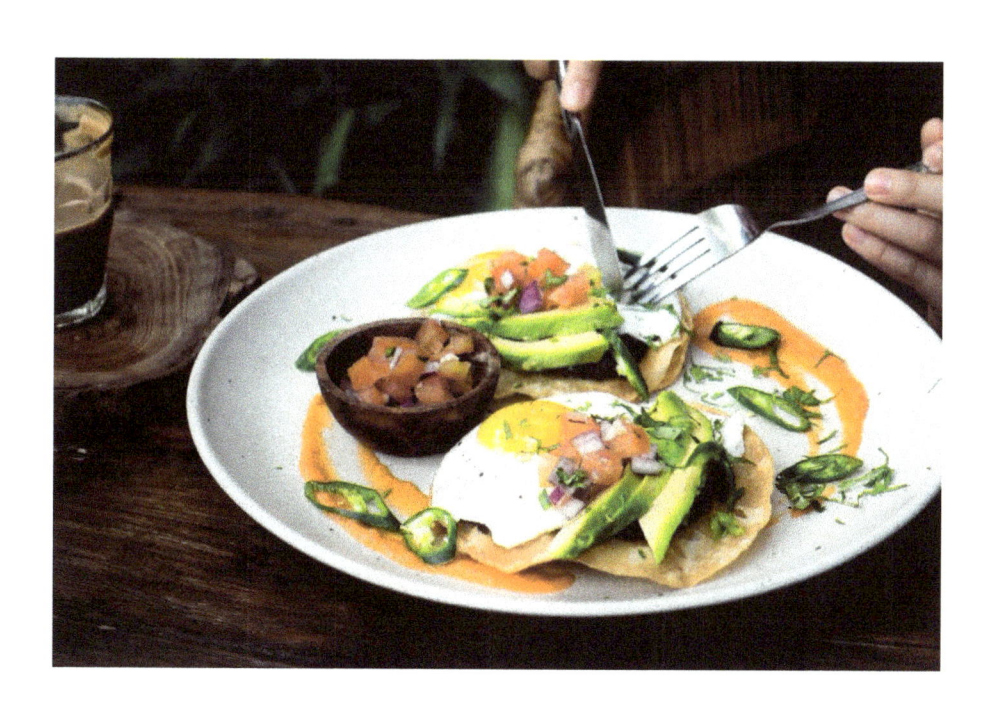

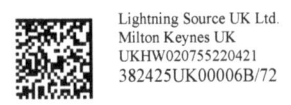